When psychologist Anne C. Bernstein's original version of *The Flight of the Stork* came out in 1978 it was well received as something innovative and helpful for those struggling to provide effective sex education for their children far beyond the stork and cabbage patch stories common to years ago. Reviewers of the original wrote...

"This is a well-conceived and well-written book, and, beyond this, an aesthetic experience. It leaves stimulating ideas hatching all over the place... To read this book is to embark on a pleasurable, enriching experience... It will be titillating if you have children of your own who are asking, and answering, and asking again the perennial question."
>Carlos Sluzki, MD, UCSF Dept. of Psychiatry
>in *Family Process*

"...some of the children's inventive ideas introduce an amusing note (but) the book is one of serious research that should prove a helpful guide to parents in gauging how much sex information their children should be given and when they should have it."
>*ALA Booklist*, April 1,1978

' (*Flight of the Stork*) is richly paced with probing interviews of children, conducted in the style of Piaget."
>Howard Gardner, author of *Frames of Mind*
>in "Getting Acquainted with Jean Piaget"
>*New York Times*, January 3, 1979

This 1994 edition brings into the 21st century the issue of what children understand about where babies come from. Today, babies come to their families through sexual intercourse, through adoption, through assisted reproductive technology, through donor insemination and surrogates, through blending of families of origin. And because of this complexity, parents need even more help. Anne C. Bernstein offers that concretely and supportively. Advance comments on the new version include...

REVISED EDITION

Flight of the Stork

REVISED EDITION

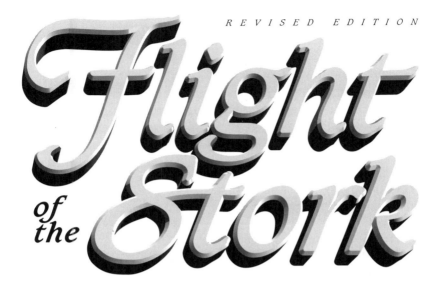

Flight of the Stork

What Children
Think (and When)
about Sex and
Family Building

Anne C.
Bernstein

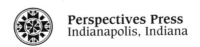

Perspectives Press
Indianapolis, Indiana

Perspectives Press
P.O. Box 90318
Indianapolis, IN 46290-0318
U.S.A.

Manufactured in the United States of America

ISBN #0-944934-09-9

Revised Edition, First printing September, 1994

Library of Congress Cataloging-in-Publication Data:

Bernstein, Anne C., 1944-
    Flight of the stork : what children think (and when) about sex and family building / Anne C. Bernstein. — Rev. ed.
        p.   cm.
    Includes bibliographical references (p.   ) and index.
    ISBN 0-944934-09-9 (pbk.) : $14.00
    1. Sex instruction for children.   2. Children's questions and answers.   I. Title.
    HQ57.B49   1994
    612.6'07—dc20   94-21672
                                                                        CIP

*D*edication

For my mother and father

Clara Handelman Bernstein and
Alfred Jacob Bernstein

*A*cknowledgments

I would like to thank the people who helped make this book possible.

I am grateful to the many readers—parents and teachers—who had continued to use *The Flight of the Stork* during the years it was out of print, encouraging me to revise and expand the original work and pursue publishing a new edition.

My son, David, and stepsons, Brian, Antonio, and Sean, gave me the opportunity to follow my own advice. Their lively curiosity and ingenious turns of mind gave me a deeper appreciation of the tasks that confront all parents. I am grateful to them for teaching me how conversations about sex and birth and forming families happen in everyday life.

Most particularly, I am indebted to Pat Johnston, noted infertility and adoption educator, and the editor and publisher of this volume. Her guidance was essential in developing the new materials, expanding the scope of the book from children's concepts of human reproduction to a broader understanding of how people form families. Most of the new material in this book addresses how children can better understand their origins when they have joined their families through adoption or have been born through assisted reproductive technologies—*in vitro* fertilization, donor insemination, ovum transfer, and surrogacy. I couldn't have done this work without Pat Johnston's inspiration and guidance.

I am also indebted to a number of other professionals, educators and advocates in the field of third party reproduction for putting me in touch with people to interview and sharing their own expertise. Fay Johnson and Shirley Zager of the Organization of Parents Through Surrogacy, Carol Frost Vercollone of RESOLVE, Inc. and Carole LieberWilkins of RESOLVE of Los Angeles County, Hillary Hanafin of the Center for Surrogate Parenting, Christie Montgomery of Surrogate Parenting Services, and Tim Fisher of the Gay and Lesbian Parents Coalition International (Washington, D.C.) all gave generously of their time and knowledge of the field. Chicago therapist Judith Calica and pediatrician and therapist Vera Fahlberg provided critiques of the new material.

Flight of the Stork found its way to Perspectives Press thanks to talented colleagues in developmental psychology. Judith Newman, a professor at Pennsylvania State University, invited me to be on a panel for a Jean Piaget Society meeting. There I met David Brodzinsky, whose research on children's understanding of adoption created the basis for Chapter 9. Without the extensive work of Brodzinsky and his colleagues, Anne Braff Brodzinsky, Marshall Schechter and Leslie Singer, I could not have addressed these issues in such depth. I am grateful to him, too, for creating the link to Pat Johnston and Perspectives Press. Johnston credits reproductive endocrinologist William R. Keye, Jr. for introducing her to the first edition when both were working as RESOLVE volunteers in Indiana in 1980.

Those who contributed to the original work must also be thanked anew. Philip A. Cowan first pointed out the need for a study of children's thinking about the origin of babies. His guidance throughout the original research was invaluable. Margaret T. Singer, Kenneth Craik, and Joseph Kuypers provided many helpful suggestions, and Sonne Lemke's work on children's identity concepts added an important dimension to the research. I am grateful, too, to Elliot Turiel for directing me toward resources to update my understanding of Piagetian theory.

The children I spoke with, and their parents, who consented to their children's being interviewed, were, of course, indispensable. The children, with their ingenuous and imaginative views and their eagerness to serve as consultants, made the work a pleasure. The Children's Community Center and the Berkwood-

Hedge School in Berkeley, California, the Early Childhood Education Department of Cabrillo College in Aptos, California, and Maria Pinedo of San Francisco all helped me make connections with children and families.

Lonnie Barbach, Ernest Callenbach, Daniel Goldstine, Katherine Larger, and David Swanger provided encouragement and assistance in the critical juncuture between completed thesis and first publication.

Donald Rothman read the manuscript as I wrote it, keeping me attentive to questions of style and clarity. An innovative teacher of writing, he more than anyone else provided both support and criticism as the first edition was in progress. Betty Cohen, Martin Gold, Alan Graubard, and Diana Rothman made many excellent suggestions for revising the first edition. Loni Hart, Nancy Feinstein, Wendy Roberts, and Vicki Strang were valuable consultants. Rhoda Weyr, my agent for the first edition, and Betty Kelly, my editor at Delacorte were vital sources of both personal and technical support. Jim Shortridge and Shelley Ross, of the SIECUS library, provided invaluable assistance in bringing my recommended resources up to date. Pat Johnston, Diane Ehrensaft, and Conn Hallinan read drafts of the new material; their editorial acumen has made for a stronger book.

I would like to single out my husband, Conn Hallinan, for special appreciation, because I especially appreciate him. A talented, creative teacher of journalism, he has become my editor of first resort, taking time from his own considerable workload to read my work "hot off the printer." His loving constancy has made all the difference.

Table of Contents

*N*otes for the *Second Edition*

Many things have changed since 1978, when *The Flight of the Stork* was first published. The birth rate has revived after a prolonged dip that led school districts to sell off empty buildings they would later find they needed. The need for sex education, both at home and at school, was amplified by the destructive consequences of not educating young people about sex. The rate of teenage pregnancy has continued to increase, and sexually transmitted diseases have become epidemic. In 1978, AIDS was unheard of, and the notion that sex could be lethal would have been dismissed as reactionary backlash to the sexual revolution. Only a few researchers were starting to open the closet door on child sexual abuse.

The need to talk with children about sex and reproduction is greater than ever. They need to know about sex to keep their curiousity alive, encouraging the lively pursuit of the answers to these and other questions. They need to know about sex to protect their health and safety. And they need to know about sex to develop satisfying, mutually respectful relationships throughout their adolescent and adult lives.

Because times have changed, some of the specific ideas children hold may change with the information they are exposed to in their family lives and in the media, but how they approach problem-solving and what they are likely to distort will follow predictable patterns. Because *Flight of the Stork* is about how children's thinking develops, the principles on which it is based continue to inform parents about what their children are likely to understand, and misunderstand, about the origin of babies.

This is a book about the origin of families, as well as the origin of babies. In thinking about how people get babies, children ponder how they happened to have the family fate has dealt them. In the original study, I asked children how do mommies get to be mommies, how daddies get to be daddies, and how do they happen to have their own particular parents. Their answers let me know that this was a question to which they had already devoted time and attention.

In the years since first publication, families have become more diverse. There are more single parent families, more families formed through adoption, more stepfamilies, and more families headed by same-sex couples. The ways all families reproduce has become more varied, thanks to innovations in medical technology that permit the creation of babies without sex. For children in families that diverge from the *Ozzie and Harriet, Father Knows Best* version of American "nuclear" family life, and for their classmates, the question "where do I come from?" cannot be answered by simply disclosing "the facts of life."

To address these concerns, I have substantially expanded *The Flight of the Stork* to address how children think about stepfamily formation, adoption and assisted reproductive technology and to help parents think through how to discuss these topics with their children. The new material is half again as long as the revised original work. In Chapter 9, I address the challenge presented to children by the still more complex concepts of *in vitro* fertilization, donor insemination, ovum transfer, and surrogracy, making suggestions to parents about how and when to discuss these topics with their children. In Chapter 10, I examine the development of children's thinking about adoption: what it means to be adopted, how they understand the motives of adoptive parents and birthparents in making an adoption plan, and their evolving understanding of the permanence of the family formed by adoption. In Chapter 11, I explore how children understand the tangle of relationships created by remarriage, when they may have a mother and a stepmother; a father and a stepfather; full, half-, and stepsiblings; and grandparents galore.

When I wrote the first edition, I had studied children's concepts of how people get babies, but I had never been called upon to put into practice the advice I had given others. In the years since, I have become a stepmother and a mother, and I have had to practice what I'd been preaching. I found that the principles on which this book is based have worked for me and my family. In thinking about how what I would say would be received by our boys at different ages, I was rewarded by having the kinds of conversations I had imagined to be possible. I hope this book gives my readers the understanding, the tools, and the confidence to do the same.

Preface

Storks fly through the air dangling babies from diaper slings. Cabbage patches are filled with infants hidden among the leaves. Doctors pull forth babies from black bags. The traditional child-tailored myths of creation are on the way out. Happily, few children are now being told these age-old parental lies, and fewer still believe them.

As part of my research at the University of California, Berkeley, I decided to find out what children understand of the explanations and gossip that form their early sex education. So I asked children their own perennial question: How do people get babies? And they told me.

It might seem as if the answer to that question will depend on what a child has been told, but that's not the case. Children continue to amaze the adults who have conscientiously imparted the "facts of life" with their own fantasized versions of these "facts." Even when adults give children straight facts, the story of human reproduction often gets twisted into a remarkable version of creation.

Jane, age four, told me, "To get a baby to grow in your tummy, you just make it first. You put some eyes on it. Put the head on, and hair, some hair, all curls. You make it with head stuff you find in the store that makes it for you. Well, the mommy and daddy make the baby and then they put it in the tummy and then it goes quickly out."

Jane had never been told that babies were manufactured, using parts purchased from the store. She put together the answer out of information pieced together by a thread of child logic that reflected her understanding of the physical world.

How did I happen to be talking to Jane about how people get babies? My interest in sex education began some years back.

In 1948, I was four years old and my mother was pregnant. My parents "prepared" me for Andrew's birth by reading to me Marie Hall Ets's book, *The Story of a Baby*. It soon became my favorite. I loved the story of the egg "smaller than a seed of hay that flies like dust in the wind" growing in its "house without windows or doors." I was fascinated by the pictures of the wrinkled, tightly curled embryos that changed from a curious squiggle on the page to something that looked just like a baby.

In those days, I could not yet read, but I could remember. I delighted in amazing adults by reciting word for word the books I had heard most often, turning the pages at the appropriate time. For the "baby book," though, I wanted an audience of children, since I was eager to share this wonderful story with my friends. I made the rounds of the neighborhood, "reading" the book to all the kids. Years later I learned that my educational campaign had caused a flood of phone calls from the other mothers to mine: "Do you know what your daughter is doing?!"

A few years after Andrew was born, I started lobbying (in vain) for a sister. My mother seemed reluctant to come right out and say that two children would do quite nicely thank you. Instead, she rested her case on a statement of fact: There was no baby growing inside her now. "Well," I argued, "just tell Daddy to plant the seed." My brother, playing nearby with a pail and shovel, came into the conversation, waving his shovel: "Me help Daddy plant the seed." I knew that was silly. Although how the seed was planted was still a mystery to me, I knew that it didn't take a shovel and was nothing a three-year-old could do.

As a child, I wanted to learn about what adults thought about having babies and what their sexual experiences were. Later, as an adult, I turned to the study of children's ideas of how people get babies. Early in my graduate studies I took a class with

Philip A. Cowan. I remember his saying that there had been much speculation about how children think about how people get babies, most of it based on adult memories or projections about childhood. While some studies collected anecdotes from children, none had systematically asked the children themselves. Years later, when I was ready to begin my own research, I decided to devote myself to this inquiry.

I talked with over a hundred children from three to twelve years old. I asked them how people get babies, how mommies get to be mommies, and how daddies get to be daddies. I asked them when mothers and fathers start to be mothers and fathers, and called upon each child to explain how <u>his</u> mother and father got to be his mother and father. I asked what the word "born" means and what had happened at the child's birth. All of the children interviewed had at least one younger brother or sister, and I asked each child why his younger sibling had come to live at his house as part of his family.

I asked the younger children: What if some people who lived in a cave in the desert, where there weren't any other people, wanted to have a baby. Because they had never known any other people, they didn't know how people get babies. What if they asked you for help? If they asked you what they should do if they wanted a baby, what would you tell them?

And to the older children, my question was: What did you think about how people get babies before you understood it as well as you do now? What did you think when you were little?

I approached each child as a consultant, asking his or her help in my work, which I explained was learning how kids think about some things. I emphasized that it was their way of think-ing, not the rightness or wrongness of their answers, that interest-ed me. I did not provide the children with any information, nor did I introduce terms or concepts not mentioned by the children them-selves. In speaking with over one hundred children, never did one turn the tables on me to ask me information about reproduction.

I use the ages of children in my examples only to help identi-fy the children speaking. These ages are not intended as norms, or indications of how a child "should" think about reproduction at age four, seven, or eleven. The sequence of the levels which I will discuss should be the same for all children, but the ages at which they are reached may differ considerably. The children I talked with are not representative of the entire population. Most, but not all, are white and middle-class. They live in a fairly sophisticated region of the country (the San Francisco Bay Area), and they have received more direct teaching on this subject than most children have. While education does not completely determine the level of explanation children give to the question "How do people get babies?" repeated experience with ideas does have an influence. As a result, we can expect that the children described in this book are probably a little younger than most of the children whose thinking about the origin of babies theirs most resembles.

Parents should not become discouraged about their children's rate of development or attempt to push them to race up the "ladder" of developmental levels. Swiss psychologist Jean Piaget calls this desire to speed up the natural rhythms of children's learning "the American disease"— racing to the end instead of enjoying the journey.

The world has become so complex that many of us find ourselves awed by the responsibility of raising children when we cannot anticipate how accelerating change will transform the conditions they will live with as adults. Our grandparents did not question that they knew what they needed to be good parents. If they had any questions, they were confident that their own parents could provide the answers. Many of the adults I know best feel that our parents did not, and could not, prepare us for the world we now live in. We are unsure about how to equip our own children to live with change and to take control over change in order that they and the world may survive.

Such uncertainty about parenting has led to an unprecedented search for experts to tell us how: how to love, how to fight, how to like ourselves, and especially, because it is part of the way we ourselves can change the world, how to raise our children. There is nothing so revealing about the true dimensions of an expert than the discovery that others look to you for advice about how to live and trust important aspects of their children's future to your counsel. In writing a book that goes beyond describing children's thinking, to suggest how to talk with them, I have been humbled by the responsibility.

And so a word about "experts" and how to use the advice they have to offer. As you cut the suit to fit your body and not your body to fit the suit, so take expert advice only when it fits. If what I suggest goes against your grain, trust yourself. You'll be a better parent for it.

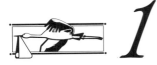

1

Children Think Differently from Adults

Alan: If Daddy put his egg in you, then
(AGE 3)   I must be a chicken.

Susan: To get a baby, go to the store and buy
(AGE 3)   a duck.

Every day, thousands of parents sit down to tell their children about the birds and the bees. And the cows. And the chickens. And the ducks. Parental descriptions of sex and birth often sound like morning roll call on Noah's ark. When it comes to people, however, the roll call becomes a lecture, taking on the precision of an advanced anatomy course, as the anxious parent rushes through enough detail to confuse a medical student.

Children take this information, process it through mental jungle gyms, and create their own versions of who comes from where, and how. The children seem content with their answers, and parents, having provided the answers, are not about to start following up with more questions. Chances are, therefore, that misunderstanding will persist.

The most effective way to tell children about sex is to provide information matched to their level of mental development. But because children aren't asked what they really believe, as opposed to what they were told, we don't understand how their ability to analyze and assimilate information changes year by year.

Do you remember what you thought as a child about how people get babies? Take a few minutes to recollect what you believed when you were four years old. Then close your eyes and come up the years to age eight. How had your understanding changed? By the time you were twelve, what did you think?

In talking with groups of parents and psychology students, I asked them to think themselves back to childhood and share their beliefs about procreation. Many find this a difficult thing to do. They find they cannot remember what their child selves believed about sex and birth. Others remember only what they were told by their parents.

One man of about thirty recalled his father explaining how you know the baby is coming long before it actually arrives. He said getting a baby was very much like going to a bakery: You go to the hospital and get a number; when your number is called, you return to collect your baby.

A woman remembered believing that to get a baby you put in a purchase order at the hospital. She had figured this out for herself and believed it until she was eleven. To put this story together, she drew on her own experience. Her father had shown her the hospital where she and her brothers and sisters were born, pointing it out to her as "the place we got all you kids." Throughout her childhood she had seen him handle countless purchase orders, since he ran his business from their home, so it was only logical that he had sent out a purchase order for them.

A woman remembered believing that a string goes from the father to the mother during lovemaking, and it is this string that impregnates her.

A man recalled his boyhood belief that intercourse was like urination and took place standing up.

A woman remembered thinking that birth occurred when the baby turned the knob of a little door in the sleeping mother's back and walked out.

An older European woman told of her fright when, having missed a period as a teenager, she was convinced that a man had impregnated her while gallantly kissing her hand.

Perhaps your memories, like these people's, are very different from your current beliefs. Perhaps you cannot remember thinking any other way than you do now. It is hard to remember that you used to reason completely differently from the way you do now. The difficulty of translating thoughts from child logic to adult logic may block the road to memory.

This book is about some of the ways that children think differently from adults. In reading these pages, adults can learn to translate some of what they know into child logic so that they may communicate better with their children. By talking with children about how people get babies, I have gathered a collection of amusing stories which beautifully illustrate the way children think. The "out of the mouths of babes" quality of many of them is touching, and the adult who listens carefully has a lot to learn.

Many parents still find it difficult to talk about reproduction with their children. Their own emotional discomfort in talking about sex is one stumbling block, and their lack of information about what the child is really asking and is likely to understand is another. I will try to present a systematic description and explanation of the ways in which children are likely to embellish fact with fable at different ages. Knowing the direction in which your children's thinking is developing can help you present information in the way they can most readily absorb. I have divided children's explanations of the origins of babies into their six levels of problem-solving ability. In Chapters 3 through 8, I will present each level: the children's ideas about how people get babies, how their theories of reproduction tie in with their ideas about other of life's puzzles, and how parents can use this insight into children's thinking to communicate more effectively with their children.

The idea that children's thinking develops through a series of levels is based on the work of Jean Piaget. Piaget regards each child as a philosopher who works at making the universe intelligible. Children ask themselves and others: What makes it night? What is a dream? How do people get babies? In growing up, children attempt to piece together answers to these and other questions, to explain to themselves the whats and hows and whys of the events that surround and involve them. They use all the resources at their disposal: what they themselves perceive with their senses, the information given them by others, and their own style of putting the puzzle together. As children develop, they shape the world in terms of their own level of understanding and then restructure their understanding when they take in information that doesn't fit into their old view of the universe. It is this structuring, restructuring, and eventual understanding that we are going to be talking about.

Piaget believed that the maturation of the nervous system and the muscular system plays a role in development, but it does not steal the show. He believed that the effect of the environment is important, but the child does not sit back passively and wait to be shaped by the outside world. Instead, Piaget emphasized, from infancy onward the child actively seeks contact with the environment, looking for new levels of stimulation. When an event occurs, it is not merely registered as a "copy" of reality, but is interpreted and assigned meaning by the child. A blanket is not a blanket is not a blanket. To one child a blanket is something to suck, to another something to hide under while playing peek-a-boo, to a third it provides warmth during sleep, and to yet another it is a source of security and good feeling to cling to when alone.

How then does the child actively move from one stage of thinking to another? As we have already noted, maturation is necessary for development, but it is not enough. The child's intellect must also interact with the world around her. Only when the external world clashes with concepts already established in her mind is the child forced to modify these concepts and develop intellectually. Piaget described this movement from stage to stage as resulting from the interaction of three different processes: assimilation (taking in), accommodation (putting out), and equilibration (balancing).

Each stage or level represents a general approach to understanding experience. Basic to Piaget's way of thinking about children's developing knowledge is that they cannot skip or leap over steps; each way of solving problems builds on the previous way. Cultural and individual differences may speed up, slow down, or even step development, so that all children of the same age are not at the same level, but the order of the levels each child must move through stays the same.

The invariance of this sequence of stages, even the very existence of stages in children's thinking, has become quite controversial in the years since Piaget stopped writing. Instead of seeing cognitive stages as basic, general, deep-seated and all pervasive, some developmental psychologists doubt that post-infancy styles of solving problems, or making sense of the world, are radically different at different ages. Part of the problem is the difficulty in accurately assessing whether qualitative shifts in solving one set of problems is truly coordinated with similar ways of thinking about very different subjects. Another is that the evidence points to slower and more gradual transitions in cognitive development rather than the abrupt step-like shifts suggested by the idea of stages.

What sense does it then make to talk about stages? In looking at children's developing cognition, it is improbable that what we are looking at is simply the uncoordinated acquisition-of-expertise in a multitude of intellectual tasks. Despite agreement that Piaget's formal model is not wholly adequate to describe the changes in children's thinking, experts in developmental psychology have judged that "some of his more informal generalizations... seem very insightful and likely to prove at least roughly correct." (Flavell, 1977, p.93) Elliot Turiel suggests that the concept of stages is still a useful one, with the proviso that transitions between them be seen as gradual rather than abrupt. In this view, development entails qualitative changes within each subject area. Transitions include a gradual process of becoming disenchanted with old ideas and then accepting new ones. For example, a child will first reject new information that does not fit with her old way of viewing the world, then begin to criticize her existing ways of thinking, and later go on to construct and maintain a more advanced set of ideas.(Turiel,1986).

In the descriptions that follow of children's thinking about how people get babies, the sequence of stages was originally thought of in Piagetian terms, although there was always an appreciation of uneven development across tasks and long periods of transition. I would also like to remind the reader that the ages given for each

level are not standards of "normality." Nor are they measures of
general intellectual development. They serve only to describe the
children I talked with whose thinking is described by that level.
To compare your children to those quoted here in order to see how
they "measure up" is to do them a disservice.

Because children are not miniature adults, they will not think
like adults until they are themselves grown up. No matter how carefully a parent explains things, a child will misunderstand some part
of the explanation, sometimes at the time, sometimes later. So, you
might ask, why put the extra effort into answering questions with
the child's thinking in mind? Why correct confusion that growing
up will straighten out anyhow?

Perhaps the most important reason is that children ask their
parents sincere questions and want and deserve truthful answers.
Not the whole truth all at once, but as much of the truth as they
request. It is not necessary to reel off explanations with all the
details of a physiology text. It is important to find out what the child
wants to know, and to do your best to satisfy his or her curiosity.
Children know when their parents are being evasive, and they begin
to wonder: Am I asking something I shouldn't? Is this something
bad to think about? and Is there something wrong with me for asking? They then quickly learn that if they really want to find out
about something, they must go somewhere else for the answers. But
children also can sense when their parents are responsive, aware of
their needs, and want to inform them. They learn that they can find
out what they want to know at home and can rely on their parents as
trustworthy sources of knowledge. When they feel assured that the
channels of communication are open, they can pace their questions
to their need to know, asking one question now and waiting to mull
over new ideas before coming back to ask for more.

Another reason to encourage children's natural curiosity about
birth is that this curiosity is the starting point for their interest in
other questions of origin, the first step toward thinking about cause
and effect. Both Freud and Piaget agree that children's inquiries into
the origins of babies make up an important step in their intellectual
development. Freud calls it "the first of the great problems of life."
Piaget says, "It is true that there will be children who ask questions

about origins before they ask them about birth but even here the question arises whether it is not an interest in birth which, thwarted and projected, is not at the root of these questions about origin." He goes on to say that "children's ideas on the birth of babies follow the same laws as their ideas in general." We will explore those ideas throughout this book. For now, it is important to note that children's questions about procreation are an early foray in their search for knowledge. Encouraging the child's unguarded questions and answering responsively also encourages the child as an active, inquisitive explorer of the world.

Contrary to the old saw, what you don't know <u>can</u> hurt you. Like the little boy who said, "If Daddy put his egg in you then I must be a chicken," children who cannot distinguish between ova, the human eggs that grow babies, and the eggs we eat for breakfast have occasion for worry. What if instead of being born they had been eaten? Imagining people as cannibals of their unborn young is disturbing. The child may refuse to eat eggs, or may eat them obediently and then feel queasy.

A six-and-a-half-year-old girl told her mother, "When I grow up, I'm not getting a daddy. And if I get a baby, I'm not going to let it out." Her belief that a baby could grow inside her body without her doing anything to set that process in motion leads to other upsetting thoughts. The idea of a baby inside who will never see the light of day, the feelings of this reluctant mother turned jailer who must keep the baby locked within her body, must no doubt cause her a great deal of worry and unhappiness. How relieved she would be to understand that if she didn't "get a daddy" no baby would begin to grow.

Among older children, vagueness and confusion about the mechanics of reproduction can lead to worry about pregnancy. Perhaps the child believes a kiss can impregnate. Or, uncertain about how the sperm gets to the egg, the child may become uncomfortable simply standing close to someone of the other sex. Adult women told me of their childhood fears that toilet seats and school benches, crowded buses and subways, might expose them to the risk of unwanted pregnancy.

Misconceptions about how people get babies can lead to conception in adolescence. Margaret Mead (who did not become pregnant until she was nearly forty) remembers her girlhood beliefs in *Blackberry Winter,* "The father's role in conception was essentially a feeding role, for many acts of intercourse were believed to be necessary to build up the baby, which was compounded of father's semen and mother's blood."

Misunderstanding can cause worry and psychological upset. Mary Jane Sherfey, in her book *The Nature and Evolution of Female Sexuality,* remembers a troubled ritual of her early adolescence. When she was twelve years old, her second-best girlfriend (whose uncle was a doctor and should know) told her that menstrual flow was really the remains of a dead baby. If you had sex, her girlfriend continued, the baby was fertilized and you got pregnant. If not, the baby died, and the menses were all that was left. She did not doubt this explanation, and it worried her:

"Most questions were ultimately answered simply, 'God made us that way.' Sad. All those dead babies! It seemed so cruel and even more so that I had to catch the few remains of my own dead baby month after month on an absorbent napkin and flush him down the toilet. I also decided that there was something wrong about God's attitude toward women. After all, He created the baby in me in the first place, and He must realize that I was forbidden to have sex and fertilize the baby until I was married (or much older). So He made the baby and then murdered it—all inside me!"

On one occasion, she ritualized her grief and feelings of loss. Carefully, she wrapped her used sanitary napkins in Christmas wrapping paper, collected them in a painted shoebox, and buried them in her back yard. Solemnly she recited the Lord's Prayer and the Twenty-third Psalm over the tiny grave, saying "Good-bye, little baby."

Many misunderstandings are harmless and easily outgrown. Others become lingering concerns. Recalled by an adult who has made the transition to untroubled maturity, they make a good story. But the child who is experiencing the worry of misconstrued realities would prefer relief now to entertaining tales later.

Sympathetic, understanding adults can help reduce the child's confusion. When children learn that their parents are open and informative about answering their questions and discussing their concerns, they have available a trusted resource to turn to in times of confusion or worry. Parents' comfort and responsiveness in talking about sex and reproduction are important prerequisites to minimizing misunderstanding. Attitude provides the ground on which effective communication can be built. Knowing how children think at different developmental stages, what concepts are likely to be difficult for them and how, helps parents to build their educational efforts on a solid foundation.

Few of the parents of the children I questioned about reproduction could predict the extent of their children's sexual knowledge. Parents of children at the lowest and highest levels of understanding predicted their offspring's answers with some accuracy. Most others assumed that their children knew a great deal more than they actually did. Many parents whose children produced fantastic versions of creation assumed that their children knew "the truth," and none anticipated the distortions that turned up.

As I talked to children of various ages, it became apparent that our present efforts at sex education often confuse children. A four-year-old boy, trying to explain how people get babies, told me, "First they were little, a duck, then they grow older into a baby." His solution seemed peculiar, but his source became clear when a four-year-old girl elaborated on a similar explanation. This little girl was explicit:

Me: How would a lady get a baby to grow in her tummy?
Susan   Get a duck. 'Cause one day I saw a book about them, and they just get a duck or a goose and they get a little more growned and then they turn into a baby.
Me: A duck will turn into a baby?
Susan: They give them some food, people food, and they grow like a baby. To get a baby, go to a store and buy a duck.
Me: How did you find that out?
Susan: I just saw, find out from this book.

Notice how literally Susan takes the idea popularized in folk wisdom: You are what you eat. A more important source of her confusion lies in the way many writers prepare books about sex and birth for children. One widely distributed book, which is recommended for children as young as three, starts with a pencil dot (to repre sent an ovum), then proceeds through the sex life of flowers, bees, rabbits, giraffes, chickens, and dogs before it reaches the human level. The evolutionary approach also reveals the hidden bias that sex is really an animal activity which can best be understood by watching animals. If we, like Pythagoras, were explaining the transmigration of the soul, then all the animals might make sense. As it is, few young children can encounter this kind of explanation without confusion.

Another writer, Selma Fraiberg, discovered a four-year-old boy who knew a sex education book by heart, but insisted that some of the woman's eggs never become babies because the daddy eats them up. "It says so in my book," he claimed, and indeed it did—in a discussion of reproduction in fish.

Both of these examples show that confusion is likely to occur when several species are included in the same introductory book. When unable to figure out a certain aspect of human reproduction, the child extrapolates details from other sections of the book. These details seem no more fantastic to him in their transposed contexts than they were as originally stated. If there was a duck on page 4 and no human baby appeared until page 10, the child searching for an explanation of how that baby comes to be might mistake the layout sequence of the book for a causal sequence in the development of the baby. Before there was a baby, there was a duck!

Other studies suggest a way out of confusion. The experience of researchers into how children think about other concepts has shown that children can expand their understanding to include ways of reasoning one level more complex than their own. Using this idea as a guide, we can reduce sex misunderstanding to a minimum.

This book presents six stages in the development of children's thinking about how people get babies. Knowing the direction in which your children's thinking is developing can help you to present information in a way that they can most readily absorb.

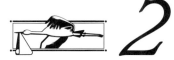

2

Talking with Your Child about Sex and Birth and Forming Families

Although children's thinking and intellectual interest in the origin of babies will be our focus, I want to avoid the all-too-common educational practice of separating sex from reproduction, emotion from physiology, personal relationship from mechanics. Too frequently, sex education is limited to diagrams and procedures, a problem in human engineering amenable to technical solutions.

But learning and knowing cannot be isolated from feeling. How I feel about myself, how I feel about my teacher, and how I feel about what I am learning all affect whether that learning will be difficult or effortless, compartmentalized or usable in other contexts.

Many educators now recognize that their classrooms are filled with feeling children, not just problem-solvers or fact memorizers. If reading, writing, and 'rithmetic skills bloom or wither depending on the emotional climate, how much more must the impact of sex education be influenced by its roots in feeling?

Only death seems to provoke the same level of discomfort most of us feel in talking about sex. Even those of us who feel some ease in talking with other adults about sex suddenly get cold feet when it's time to talk with children. Perhaps our awareness of the negative messages about sex we ourselves received as children reminds us that we need to be careful not to pass on our conflicts. Lacking real-life models for how to talk more openly with children, it is not easy to put our good intentions into action.

Whatever our feelings about sex are, we cannot avoid communicating them to our children. In addition to the verbal messages we are aware of sending, there are layers of simultaneously broadcast signals that qualify what we are trying to say. Tone of voice, inflection, facial expression, and gesture all communicate how we feel about what we are saying. Parents who tell their child that it is all right for her to masturbate, their voices flat and controlled, are giving her a double message. Their words say one thing, but the way they say it lets her know that on a deeper level they believe just the opposite. She cannot help but feel that she is doing something wrong, but because they do not acknowledge the nonverbal message, she is left confused about why she feels as she does.

Parents who evade issues, changing the subject when a question is asked or distracting the child when his behavior becomes overtly sexual, are also communicating their feelings to the child. No answer is also an answer. The message is clear if not explicit: This is something we don't talk about in this house; You are asking me improper questions I don't want to hear. The child learns that there is something wrong with him, feels embarrassed, and remains ignorant or seeks answers from friends who may know less but don't make him feel ashamed.

In *Between Marriage and Divorce*, Susan Braudy gives an example of how powerful nonverbal messages can be, leading to firmly held, but erroneous, convictions. Growing up, she never discussed either sex or religion with her mother. Instead, "my mother handed me a series of illustrated booklets about sex, when I was twelve. She had her 'I'm uneasy so don't ask' look on her face. When I was eight and asked her if she believed in God, she got that strained look on her face and told me that it was her private business. Once I found a Tampax and asked her what it was. She got the same look on her face and said nothing. So that's why I knew Tampax had something to do with religion."

While reading a book cannot provide an instant solution, the more aware we can become about our sexual values and feelings, the more informed we are on the issues, the better able we will be to teach our children about sex in an open, loving, and supportive way.

Any exchange between two people makes a statement about their relationship. A child who asks "How do you go about having a baby?" or "Does it hurt when the sperm hits the egg?" tells you that you are someone he trusts to give him reliable information without making him feel bad for wanting to know. Direct, honest responses to children's sexual curiosity give them both needed information and validation that they are good people, whose explorations of life, pleasure, and love are a valuable part of their development.

There is no way for parents to totally control the sex education of their children. I doubt whether it was ever possible, but in today's "global village" of rapid communications media, no child exposed to the light of day can be insulated from messages about sex. Not being able to control the whole show should not, however, discourage parents from assuming leading roles in the drama. Amid the clamor of competing claims to children's attention on sexual matters, there need to be reliable and loving people on whom they can depend through their years of growth. No matter what others say, they need to know what their parents think and feel about the things they are learning and feeling. Parents who establish themselves early in their children's lives as open and comfortable in dealing with sexuality will find that when their children have questions or worries to be cleared up, they will turn to their parents.

Teaching about sexuality begins at birth. The touching and handling and caressing loving parents provide in the course of infant care is essential to the newborn's survival and development. Gentle, loving touch teaches infants to relate warmly to others, while touch deprivation leads to emotional and physical problems. Studies of infants in orphanages who were fed and kept clean but deprived of adequate cuddling show how important the stimulation of skin contact can be. The institutionalized children became depressed, and their developing speech, motor coordination, and relations with others were retarded or arrested. Colds and common childhood diseases were fatal in a surprising number of cases. (Gadpaille.)

This early stimulation between parent and child, so essential for the infant's survival and growth and so different from the genital eroticism of mature adults, is nonetheless sexual. Sensual pleasure, the exchange of affection, physical closeness leading to emotional intimacy, all are there. Through early experiences of skin touching skin, infants learn whether the life of the body and physical contact with others yields pleasure or discomfort, reassurance or rejection.

Children first experience love, both giving and receiving, with their parents. So by loving children you are providing sex education, too. Children value themselves when they feel valued by the people they most love, the people on whom they know their survival rests: their parents. From their parents, children learn either "I am a lovable person whom others will care for" or "I am unlovable and must protect myself from caring too much for anyone."

The young child values his waste products as part of his body. If he is made to feel that his bowel movement or urine is bad, he may internalize these attitudes, and start to feel that he himself is bad. Similarly, children who discover that the genitals that give them pleasure cause disgust in their parents will often feel that their genitals are bad, their feelings are wrong, and they are unworthy as people. (Fraiberg.)

Long before children enter school, their gender identity and feelings about sexuality have been shaped by early experiences with family members. Feeling good about one's sexual identity is an important part of self-esteem. To like the fact of one's own sex, one must feel good about one's genitals. It is hard for a child to feel good about himself if his parents would have preferred him to have been put together differently.

In learning about sex differences, children learn both facts and values. Listening to the answers to their questions about genital differences, they pick up attitudes as well as information. Once they can move around well enough to observe others' bodies, have a social setting such as a nursery-school bathroom that permits repeated opportunities for looking, and have the mental ability to make comparisons, children will explore this intriguing discovery.

Until they see evidence to the contrary, both sexes assume that everybody is "just like me." Seeing the body of a naked child of the other sex will stimulate questions about why there's a difference. Boys may ask, "Where's her penis?" or "Why doesn't she have one, too?" or "What happened to it?" From girls, the questions may be "What is that?" or "Why does he have that?" or "What happened to mine?" Warren Gadpaille, who argues that the theory of "penis envy has been grossly misused as a basis for a thoroughly mistaken and derogatory theory of female inferiority," points out that these questions are most frequently asked "with strong curiosity but with little or no anxiety."

Unless complicated by negative attitudes toward the little girl's sexuality, penis envy is frequent but harmless. "Every parent has observed," writes Gadpaille, "and certainly every child 'knows,' that having something is preferable to not having it . . . On this basis alone, penis envy is both understandable and transient." Teaching more about other sex differences is often useful when children first begin to ask questions about genitals. The development of breasts or facial hair, changes in the size of genitals with maturation, and the presence of the female's internal organs round out the picture so that each sex is defined by what it has rather than by what it lacks. It is difficult for the girl, as well as the boy, to ask questions about something they cannot see. But both need to understand that they are specially designed, "on purpose," to be different so that they can make babies together when they are grown up.

One part of teaching is labeling. Middle-class Americans have tended to teach their children that a boy has a penis and a girl has a vagina. While clearly preferable to referring to genitals with a non-specific "down there," the word *vagina* is usually used inaccurately to refer to the female external genitals, the vulva. Until recently, the clitoris was entirely ignored by parents teaching body parts to children, leaving their daughters to discover for themselves this unlabeled part that exists only to provide pleasure.

There is no way to satisfactorily teach female anatomy if a direct equivalence must be made to the male. Alix Shulman attempts to redress past grievances by introducing new terms and concepts to the dialogue between parent and child:

Boy: What's the difference between boys and girls?

Mother: Mainly their sex organs. A boy has a penis and a girl has a clitoris.

Boy: What's a clitoris?

Mother: It's a tiny sensitive organ on a girl's body about where a penis is on a boy's body. It feels good to touch, like your penis...

Boy: What's it for?

Mother: For making love, for pleasure. When people love each other, one of the ways they show it is by caressing one another's bodies, including their sex organs.

Boy: How do girls pee?

Mother: There's an opening below the clitoris for peeing. A man uses his penis for peeing, for making love, and for starting babies. Women have three separate places for these (and so on....)

There is a great deal to applaud in this approach: using the child's curiosity as a guide in providing information; giving simple, direct answers that make the lesson a dialogue instead of a lecture; recognizing the importance of teaching boys as well as girls about female anatomy; and including talk about pleasure and lovemaking in discussing sex with children. But her comparisons are not wholly accurate. Women do not have two separate places for lovemaking and starting babies. Women and men make love with their whole bodies. While the clitoris is uniquely designed for pleasure, women's sexual preferences, as well as their patterns of genital nerve endings, do vary. We should not banish the vagina from the arena of love and pleasure to make up for the prior exclusion of the clitoris.

Children learn about sexuality as they are taught about sex differences and reproduction. For better or for worse. Rebecca Black, a San Francisco sex therapist, describes in these terms the double message parents too frequently communicate to their children: "Sex is dirty—save it for someone you love." Gadpaille urges, and I with him, "that nothing be taught to a child that he must subsequently unlearn for effective adulthood." Children taught that it is bad to pursue sexual pleasure often find it a difficult if not impossible task to convince themselves as adults that now at last it is good.

"The walls have ears," I remember groups of adults saying, drawing one another's attention to the fact that children were present, soaking up all that was said, things that were presumably over their heads. Children are observant. Noticing how adults treat each other and how they themselves are treated by adults, they are quick to catch the discrepancies between what we say and what we do, and are more deeply impressed by practice than by words. If they see that they themselves are treated with respect and are expected to be responsible to others, respecting their desires, they will come to value themselves and others, rejecting force or exploitation in their human relationships. By watching their parents' marriage, they learn how sexual intimates relate. Is the love between a woman and man mutually supportive, caring, tender, responsive, and responsible, or exploitative, critical, barren, and debasing? What they see at home as children will influence their expectations of what is possible for them when they become sexually active adults.

What a challenge. We cannot avoid communicating about sex to children. The way we relate to one another and how we talk about sexual differences, reproduction, and relationships all form a part of their sex education. How then can we guide them in their effort to integrate their sexuality into their lives as whole people when this is a task very much in progress for most of us? In order to help the children we love, we must first explore our own feelings about sexuality and become more comfortable with them. We know that a lot was lacking in our own sex education, and all of us still have some conflicts from time to time. To be clear with children we must first be clear with ourselves, recognizing that we have abilities and limits, and acknowledging our true values.

It is not always easy to talk about sex with children. Feeling ignorant is often a problem for parents. Nothing can impress us with how little we know more than a child wanting to know the hows and whys of things we have come to take for granted. How does a car work? Why does it rain? How come the sperm and the ovum have to get together to make a baby?

Luckily for most of us, you don't need to have every piece to the puzzle to get the picture across. It isn't necessary to understand all the complexities of sexual reproduction to teach your children what they want to know. Their learning, like our own, will continue throughout their lives. If you don't know the answer to a child's question, admit it and go look it up. As a fallible human being you will be more approachable than the omniscient giants we sometimes expect ourselves to be.

And "mistakes" can be remedied. If this discussion makes you feel that there are things you would like to have done differently, it is probably not too late. Attitudes, once instilled, can yet be changed. Elizabeth Canfield, prominent sex-educator, suggests, "It's a marvelous experience to walk up to a child and be able to say 'You know, I've done some more thinking about our discussion the other day and I've decided what I said didn't make sense (or it was a bunch of baloney, or garbage), so let's talk about it some more.' A child (or friend, neighbor, student, employee, lover) will be so delighted with this admission of your ability to blow it now and then, that a whole new world of communication will have opened up!"

One way for you to become more comfortable about talking about sex with children is to practice with adults. Share with your spouse or friends the questions you anticipate your child asking before they arise. Try out different ways of answering each question and then talk about which seem to fit best with your values and what you want for your child. You can take turns role-playing child and parent, giving each a turn to ask the questions a child might ask. After the "adult" in the pair responds to the "child's" questions, the "child" can report how it felt to be on the receiving end of the explanations offered, and the "adult" can share how it felt to be faced with these questions and to answer as he did. If first tries are not satisfactory, run the scene through again until you find an approach with which you are comfortable. Most people find that simply saying aloud words and phrases they had formerly only thought to themselves makes it easier to discuss sex.

Another deterrent to parents talking about sexuality with their children is the all-too-common belief that information equals permission. Not wanting to "put ideas in their heads," parents often behave as if the less their children know about sex, the better it will be for all concerned. This misguided protection is based on a false assumption. Children will have sexual feelings and interests whether or not adults acknowledge their children's sexuality. Sexual curiosity begins in the first months of life. Parents may be embarrassed or repressive about children's sexual behavior, but they cannot eliminate it without creating feelings which will handicap those children when they are grown up.

Information and knowledge do not cause damage, but secrecy and ignorance may. "No young girl was ever ruined by a book" is an old joke. But it is also true. Socially inappropriate behavior is more often the result of ignorance than of knowledge. None of us, child or adult, does everything we know to be possible. Nor do we want to. But when we know the score, we can choose which tune to sing, fitting the song to the scene and the characters with whom we share the platform.

Children need to know that they are not bad or unworthy because they are sexually curious about the bodies of others and have found sexual pleasure in their own bodies. But this does not mean that permission must extend to whatever they feel like doing with whomever they feel like doing it with. Parents can set limits on behavior without devaluing the child or his feelings. "I know you want to take your clothes off now, but when we're in the front yard I want you to wear your shorts," for example, establishes the parent's right to set limits without shaming the child or disparaging her feelings. If she then asks why, a parent may explain that there are times and places for being dressed or undressed and that front yards are one of the places where people have agreed that it is good manners to wear clothes.

Worrying about saying it just right sometimes stops parents from starting sexual discussions with children. Convinced that the right words are very important, they weigh each phrase, signaling to the children that the terrain is made of eggshells and can be approached only on tiptoes. Although their caution is exaggerated and probably defeats their intent of giving clear information, the words we choose do have an impact. Having the appropriate words enables children to understand the world, organize their thoughts, and behave in ways that make life with other people possible.

Adults often deliberately confuse children about sex. Because of their own discomfort, or convinced that the children "are too young to really understand," they use words that cloud rather than clarify the topic. Gadpaille mentions three ways that parents "contribute to childhood ignorance and confusion": by negative labeling, nonlabeling, and mislabeling.

We have already touched on negative labeling. Told that what he is doing is bad by a parent who sees his behavior as sexual, the child learns that he is bad, without being clear about what behavior is being criticized or what is wrong with It. How can he then not feel confused and anxious?

Not giving a child a vocabulary for sexuality is nonlabeling. Scolding or spanking a child who supposedly crosses the line of acceptable sexual behavior without telling her what she has done to warrant this, or distracting her from masturbating by offering another activity or physically interfering without comment, falls into this category. The result is that the child is left without the verbal building blocks to form positive sexual values.

"Finally," writes Gadpaille, "there is mislabeling. A child may be warned about supposedly harmful effects unrelated to the specifically sexual aspects of a particular behavior. For example, a masturbating girl may be told that she can hurt herself up inside. It is the sexual act that the adult wants to stop, but he mislabels it as physically dangerous, thus contributing to the child's misconception of sex as violent and harmful. Any false information, such as 'God put the seed in Mama's belly,' is mislabeling. Another form of mislabeling is the early identification of the sex organ by use of nursery or baby talk words which, in their initial application, refer to excretory functions. These words often are never replaced with sexually accurate words, and constitute a form of mislabeling that fosters the association between sexuality and dirtiness."

We don't need a lot of esoteric knowledge to avoid these pitfalls of language misuse. Rather than expertise, it requires a respect for the child's emotional and intellectual needs and the willingness to take responsibility for one's own feelings and demands. By saying "I know it feels good to touch your clitoris [or vulva], but it makes me uncomfortable when you do it in the kitchen, where I need to work; I would feel better if you would go to another room where you can have some privacy," a parent communicates his feelings and the limits he would like to place on the child's behavior without either mystifying or criticizing the child.

Although reproduction is more frequently and more easily discussed between parents and children than sexuality, many parents wonder when to tell their children about how people get babies. My opinion is that the child's own curiosity most often lets parents know when he wants information. When parents are reasonably comfortable responding to questions about sex and birth, and the environment is one in which babies are born to family, friends, or neighbors, children will ask for explanations of where and how these new additions came to he. Mother's pregnancy is, of course, the most interesting, promising the most upheaval in the child's own life. Even children whose circle of family and friends includes few births will begin to wonder about their own origins, asking where they were when Mommy and Daddy were in high school or visiting Mexico years before.

While the child's own curiosity can usually be a guide to the explicitness of your explanation, there are times when a parent should raise the topic without waiting to be asked. Too frequently parents wait for children to ask questions about sex while hoping that they won't. Fear of showing her feelings or lack of parental encouragement may underlie a child's supposed disinterest. Perhaps previous questions have been shrugged off by embarrassed parents who assumed that there would be plenty of time to deal with the subject when the child was older. Instead of taking advantage of an opportunity to casually provide simple, clear explanations, they may inadvertently have discouraged further questions.

When a child seems disinterested, parents can give him permission to express his questions by saying "When I was your age I used to have a lot of questions about sex. Do you?" A loud "No" may mean that the child needs some time to get used to talking about a previously avoided subject, and should not he taken as the final word on the matter. Many opportunities occur in daily life to discuss sex and babies casually, without the pomp and ceremony of come here-I-have-something-important-to-tell-you.

If a child notices that a school friend now has a new sibling, or a family pet has a litter, a parent may ask, "Do you know how people get babies?" If the child appears to want to know, this can be followed up with other questions until the child's level of understanding is clear, indicating where the parent needs to fill in missing pieces of the puzzle. Values as well as facts can be communicated in this way. The pregnancy of a teacher, aunt, or neighbor can provide an opportunity to discuss your feelings about having children by choice when parents are ready to take care of their young.

Once the subject has been raised, whether by you or by your child, the next important step is to find out what the child really wants to know. It is far better to tell your children what they want to know in terms they can understand than to inundate them with information. You will need to ask questions to find out what your child is really asking you. Lonnie Barbach tells of one three-and-a-half-year-old who "asked Diane, 'How does a car work?' Diane's mind immediately raced to all the complexities of a combustion engine. . . . But before she jumped in over both their heads, Diane asked, 'How do you think it works?' 'Well, I don't think you push it with your feet,' the child answered. This greatly simplified Diane's problem as she explained the absolute rudiments of a motor attached to the wheels which causes the car to move."

There's an old joke that makes the same point: Five-year-old Johnny comes home and asks his mother, "Where did I come from?" His flustered but well-meaning mother launches into a long explanation of reproduction, including sexual intercourse and conception. Impatiently, Johnny interrupts her, protesting, "I know all that. But Jimmy says he comes from Detroit. Where do I come from?"

Responding to the child who asks, "Where do babies come from?" with "What do you think?" lets you know what the child knows or guesses. Questions like these reveal misinformation or troublesome fantasies the child may be having. They prepare the ground for parents' answers, which may then be geared to the child's level of comprehension.

Never make children feel stupid or foolish because they look at reproduction in a fanciful way. Don't be afraid to let them know that you enjoy the inventiveness of their imagery. You can support children's problem-solving efforts without confirming their erroneous impressions. For example, to a child who answers "the mommy swallows a seed" to the question of how babies get started, a parent might respond, "I can see why you might think that. Most things that go in our bodies go first through our mouths, when we eat." She would then go on to explain that the baby grows in a special place called the uterus, not in the stomach, and that this special place has entrances and exits separate from those to and from the stomach. Sometimes children's words may seem like nonsense to an adult, but they do have meaning for the child. Listening respectfully to what they have to say, putting their remarks in the context of what is happening in their lives—immediate events or timely themes—reveals the underlying meaning of their comments.

You will probably he surprised by some of what your children tell you. In Chapters 3 through 8, we will look in detail at what children at different levels of comprehension do think about how people get babies. Most of the parents of the children I interviewed could not predict their offspring's responses to my questions, consistently overestimating their children's level of understanding. One mother who read an article I had published in *Psychology Today* later told me, "I said to myself, 'Oh, my kids wouldn't think anything that silly.'" So she went home and asked her nine and eleven-year-olds what they were thinking, and was surprised to hear that the nine-year-old said he was guessing and the eleven-year-old had not long ago abandoned a theory involving a long line of blue and pink bassinets. "And I thought these kids had been told all this stuff," she reported to me. "It really made me realize that children don't quite get things the way you thought they would when you told them. It was really amazing to me." She was also pleased to find that her fifth-grader, who had previously avoided all talk of sex, followed up on her opening the subject by bringing her questions he had about films in the school's sex-education program.

Learning what children are thinking helps adults make sure the foundation for understanding is sound before going on to build elaborate explanations. But it is not enough to answer their questions with questions. The child who is asked only "Well, what do you think about that?" and is given no further information will get

the message that parents are not willing to share their own knowledge and feelings. Before long. he will stop bringing his questions
to those who evade answering.

While there is no way of avoiding all misunderstanding, some
ways of presenting information are less confusing than others. It is
so much better to have a dialogue with your child than to lecture
without checking out what he or she is doing with the information
you provide. The dialogue might begin, "Well, how do you think it
happens?" A parent would then validate the child's problem-solving
effort, confirm what was accurate in the child's account, clear up or
sort out confusing threads, and then find out what it is the child
wants to know more about. Children often know their own limits,
deciding to forgo some information until they have processed what
they already know. One woman, responding to her daughter's
expressed uneasiness about birth, asked her, "Would you like me to
tell you more about what it's like?" And the girl said, "No." "I have
all I can deal with at the moment" came across without being said.

Do not be discouraged if your child comes to you with a question you thought you had answered long ago. Being told something
once is not enough for a child to learn, whether it is about sex or
geography or friendship. Children seem to need repetition to firmly
implant new concepts in their previous understanding of the world.
As they work toward ever more complex integrations of the same
subject matter, from time to time they may feel confused.

Maturation is not a steady progression of acquiring stable and
permanent abilities. "Two steps forward and one step back" probably
best describes how it feels to make gains, backslide, and gain again,
perhaps more easily the next time. This regression to earlier ways
 of behaving or thinking about the world is a normal part of development. As development proceeds. children will reevaluate and discard
former misconceptions, organizing past learning to include present
experience. To do this successfully, they need parents to give them
emotional support, the security that permits exploration. It is easier
to venture forth into unknown territories when we know that we
can touch home base when we need to.

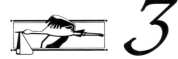

3

The Geographers–
Level One

Level One children believe that babies have always existed. These children range in age from three to seven. They are likely to answer the question How do people get babies? as if it were a question about geography. Their only problem is accounting for the whereabouts of babies before they arrive at the family hearth. They typically choose three locations for the storage of babies prior to birth. Based on their own experience getting new things, they may assume babies are bought in stores. Or perhaps the purchase takes place at the hospital. If they have been told that God arranges the arrival of babies, they may picture "God's place" as a heavenly hacienda or cloud-soft nursery. Most often, though, because of their own observations or what they have been told by parents, they think of the baby as in the mother's body before birth. Several parents have told me about their toddlers looking under mama's skirt to see the baby, untucking her blouse in further search when earlier explorations did not reveal the baby they had been told was there.

These children also believe that all children become grownups and all grown-ups are mom-

mies and daddies. As babies begin to grow automatically, as part
of the maturational process, so all girls grow to be mommies and
all boys become daddies. They may even be mommies and daddies
without having children. But if they do not as yet have children, that
is just a matter of time. If they eat their vegetables and want babies
enough, they will have them. And to not want babies is, to these
young children, unthinkable. Nurturing babies and little children is
as important and as valuable as any human activity. It means minis-
tering to them.

Whether informed or misinformed by parents and friends,
children's thinking about how people get babies will depend on their
problem-solving ability. How they think will mold what they think.
They will listen to others' accounts, adopting some, discarding some,
in their efforts to reconstruct their own version of creation.

As adults, we often take for granted concepts that children can
only learn gradually. In thinking about the origin of babies, children
begin to grapple with two concepts integral to the unraveling of life's
mysteries: identity and causality.

Identity

However much my appearance may have changed as I grew
and matured, my identity is constant and my sense of self is con-
served despite the transformations I may see in my mirror over the
years. It is only when I recognize that you and I are the same people
we have always been that I can think about my own origins and
those of my brothers and sisters.

Jimmy is three years old. After our interview his mother handed him some of his baby pictures for him to show me. He looked at
a picture of himself taken two years earlier and said, "That's Mikey."
Mikey, his younger brother, closely resembled the infant in the
picture. Anyone might have made the same mistake. His mother corrected him, "I know it looks like Mikey, but that was you when you
were a baby." And Jimmy asked, "That was me when I was Mikey?"

Sparky is a young brown-and-white pony. He lives in the yard
of a nursery school. One day Marsha, the nursery school teacher,

brought in a picture of herself as a four-year-old seated on a brown-and-white pony. And all of the children asked, "Is that Sparky you're riding?"

For these youngsters, appearance is all-important in determining identity. We can imagine that children's thinking goes something like this: If I used to look just like my brother perhaps I used to be my brother. If the brown-and white pony I ride at age four looks just like the pony my teacher rode when she was four, it must be the same pony.

Young children asked to identify each member of a large family in a series of photographs begin by denying the identity of anyone who does not look exactly alike in both pictures. If a child has changed dresses or cut her hair, they will reject the possibility that she is the same person. They cannot discriminate between the essential and the inessential aspects of who's who. A little later they will base their identifications on more ephemeral things: "He's the same boy because he's got straight hair" or "because he's got sunglasses," "She's the same girl because she has a pretty dress" or "because she's got curly hair." (Lemke) Identities can be handed down with used clothing.

It is not until they are six or seven that children let go of the belief that magical transformations are possible. In a study by Lawrence Kohlberg, most four-year-olds said that a girl could be a boy if she wanted to, or if she played "boy games", or if she wore a boy's hair style or clothes. They also claimed that a cat could be a dog if it wanted to, or if its whiskers were cut off. By six or seven, most children were insistent that neither cat nor girl could change species or sex regardless of changes in appearance or behavior. They had learned that identity is permanent and cannot be disrupted by apparent transformations.

Causality

As children learn to conserve identity, they are also developing the concept of causality. It is only when children begin to perceive that events and phenomena have causes that they can attempt to investigate what those causes are. It is not immediately obvious that today's events may be related to yesterday's deeds that made them happen. To be able to accurately link two activities in a "because" statement, children must first explore the relationships that are most noticeable and pertinent to them.

The same child who tells you that one boat floats "because it's red" may tell you that another floats "because it's blue" or "because it's big." Size and color are the boat's most outstanding features. Therefore, the child feels that floating must be explainable by these very apparent dominant characteristics.

A little later, children are less random in their explanations. Instead, the world becomes a utopia organized by the people for the people. Children explain origins in psychological or moral language. Night falls so that we may go to sleep, and trees grow so that we may eat fruit. I cannot watch Ellen's dreams because she doesn't want me to see them. Cows moo because they don't want to talk people talk. And children have the mommies and daddies they do because those were the parents they wanted.

As we explore the different levels of children's thinking about the origin of babies, we will see how their concept of causality develops from these primitive beginnings to an understanding in harmony with the Western scientific thought that dominates our culture.

Level One. Geography

The youngest children answered the question, "How do people get babies?" as if it were a question about geography. These children, usually three to five years old, told me:

"You go to a baby store and buy one."

"You get babies from tummies."

"Babies come from God's place."

"It just grows inside Mommy's tummy. It's there all the time. Mommy doesn't have to do anything. She just waits until she feels it."

These children assume that babies, like themselves and all those who people their world, have always existed. The problem is only to discover where the baby was before it came to live wherever it is now.

A "Dennis the Menace" cartoon captures the essence of the child's assumption that he has always existed. The illustration shows Dennis and his parents in a darkened room, watching a home movie. On the screen, his parents, dressed in tuxedo and wedding gown, are being showered with rice by smiling people as a minister waves good-bye. The caption has Dennis complaining, "I suppose I was home with the sitter while all this was goin' on."

How can the world have existed before he did? How can his parents, in whose lives he is so prominent, have lived without him? Toys exist because he plays with them. His dog Ruff is there because Dennis loves him. Mother makes it night by turning out the light so that he can go to sleep. A world so clearly organized around him could not have preceded him. The egocentrism of the young child leads him inevitably to the conclusion that he must have always existed. A world without him is inconceivable.

But all these other babies. They weren't always here. Each child remembers a time when some younger child was not around. Where did she come from? Where did they get him? Children hear stories about their own birth, about the time before they were in their family, and can only conclude that they must have been some place else. Where then?

Children typically think of one of three places in trying to account for where babies were warehoused before birth.

Nine Pounds Four Ounces at $10 a Pound

"Mommy bought me in a shop," a four-year-old boy told Piaget sixty-five years ago. Several of the children I talked with recently made the same claim. Since almost everything new that comes into their lives is bought, new babies must also come from a store.

Nina told me, "Babies come from their houses. You can buy some babies in somebody's house." She is four.

Dick, nearly four, would give this advice to people who wanted to be parents, "First you has to go to a baby store and buy a baby." I asked him, "Have you ever seen a baby store?"

Dick: No.

Me: Do you think there are some?

Dick: Yeah. Yeah, way far away. Right up there. From the hill.

Me: And people go there?

Dick: Yeah. I went there yesterday, and I saw babies. I heard them cry but I didn't even look at them. I just heard them cry. So I think you buy one if it cries, if you don't want him to cry you just have to put his head on his stomach and that means he doesn't cry any more. Yeah, that's how you buy a baby.

Grant, just three, claims to have seen such a store. I asked him how people get babies. "Buy them," he said, "from the baby store." Had he seen such a store? "Yeah." But were there babies there? "Yeah, our sister. She was sleeping on a shelf."

Grant, like Dick, was redecorating his memory to match his experience that new acquisitions come from commercial transactions. But, with an egalitarian flair, Grant sees children as consumers as well as goods in the family marketplace.

Me: How come Laurie's your mommy?

Grant: Cause that's my mom, and dad.

Me: How come?

Grant: Cause I wanted them. Tara [his sister] and me buyed them. I buyed a daddy and Tara buyed a mommy.

This turnabout, asserting that it is children who choose their parents rather than parents who arrange to have children, denies the very real imbalance of power between adults and their preschool children and illustrates the weight children give to their own wishes.

The Heavenly Nursery

Another popular location for storing babies prior to their arrival at the family hearth is "God's place." Few of the children I talked with believed that babies were "bundles from heaven." Instead, they located unborn infants in their mother's bodies or in the market-place. I imagine, however, that in communities where religion plays a more influential role in people's lives, parents' teaching that babies are a gift from God would satisfy the curiosity of the preschooler, who requires only a geographical location to account for the origin of babies.

Many adults have told me that their early childhood beliefs resembled greeting-card cartoons of birth: hundreds of babies lolling around on clouds, passing the time in friendly play until it comes time to be taken, by stork or heavenly messenger, to their waiting parents.

Mommy's Body

Alexandra will soon be four. She told me that a baby "just grows inside Mommy's tummy. It's there all the time. Mommy doesn't have to do anything. She just waits until she feels it." We continued to talk:

Me: How did your brother start to be in your mommy's tummy?

Alexandra: Um, my baby just went in my mommy's tummy.

Me: How did he go in?

Alexandra: He was just in my mommy's tummy.

Me: Before you said that he wasn't there when you were there. Was he?

Alexandra: Yeah, and then he was in the other place... In America.

Me: In America?

Alexandra: Yeah, in somebody else's tummy. And then he went through somebody's vagina, and then he went in my mommy's tummy.

Me: In whose tummy was he before?

Alexandra: I don't know who his—her name is. It's a her.

For this little girl, typical of the Level One children, a baby that now exists must always have existed. The only real question is where he was before he came to live at her house. She knows that her brother grew inside her mother's body. The question of how and when he started to grow there are beyond her grasp at the moment, but she extrapolates from the information she has: Babies grow inside tummies and come out vaginas. If there was a time prior to her brother's being in her mother's tummy, then he must have been in some place else, in somebody else's tummy, and that somebody else must be female, because "only big girls can grow babies in their tummies." Presumably this chain can go on indefinitely, with each mommy getting her baby in turn from another woman.

Penny, too, sees a baby as a gift that is passed around until it is finally given to its mother. I asked her, "How do people get babies?"

Penny: My mommy does. She gets babies.

Me: How?

Penny: She gets her baby from Bill (Penny's father). From Peggy.

Me: How does Peggy get the baby?

Penny: She got it from Peter (who gets it) from Danny (who gets it) from me.

Me: How did you get the baby?

Penny: From my dad.

Me: From your dad? How did that happen?

Penny: I got it from my mother, my big sister. Well, my sister's name is Lisa. Well, next Mommy got from Lisa.

Most of the children saw no need to string together a series of locations for the baby before birth. If the baby grows inside its mommy's body, then it must always have been there. Alexandra was dislodged from her initial belief that babies were always in mommies' tummies by being called to account for her brother's whereabouts when she was in their mother's tummy. Jacob felt no need to resort to geographical guesses about his sister. Quite willing to share the occupancy of their mother's body, he told me joyfully, "Tina and I were in the womb together. We were hugging in the womb."

Most of these children were either unenlightened or had forgotten that there was a special place for babies to grow inside Mommy.

They told me the baby grows in Mommy's tummy or stomach. A few, however, described babies as coming from Mommy's breasts. Three-year-old Sandra told me people get babies "out of geegees (breasts)."

Sandra: Like this, they come out (waving her arm away from her chest). They've got to get milk in the geegees then. Babies come out of geegees.

Me: Whose geegees do they come out from?

Sandra: Everybody's.

Me: Do they come out of yours?

Sandra: When I grow up.

For the children of nursing mothers, babies and breasts are as strongly linked as peanut butter and jelly. Since only women have developed breasts and only women grow babies, breasts must figure prominently in the origins of babies. An anthropological parallel is found among the Sinaupolo aborigines, who believe conception takes place in the breasts since these first show signs of the women's condition.

I continued to question Sandra:

Me: Do babies come out of daddies' geegees?

Sandra: Noooooo.

Me: Mommies'?

Sandra: Yes.

Me: Why don't they come out of daddies?

Sandra: Because their body has hair.

A few children thought that girl babies come from mommies and boy babies come from daddies, presumably based on the principle that "like begets like," with each parent reproducing his or her own kind of person. But this response was uncommon. When asked if babies grow in daddies' tummies, and if not, why not, most children at this level stated "they just don't" without being able to explain why. Others, like Sandra, focus on an easily observable sex difference that bears no obvious connection to childbearing. Three-year-old Penny based her conclusion on daddies' inability to feed the baby "because daddies got little nipples and mommies got big nipples." Jeff, who is four, told me, "Babies come out of mommies' tummies. They just crawl through the tunnel. Daddies just don't have tunnels like mommies do," so, of course, babies cannot grow in their tummies. His success in making a causal link builds on his accurate grasp of anatomy.

The characteristic limitation of all children at this first level, however accurate their understanding of basic anatomy, is their inability to account in any way for the baby's beginning to grow in its mother's body. Penny's response is typical: "They just grow inside. I don't know how it starts. It just grows." When queried further, they fall back on one of two sets of assumptions: Babies are in girls' tummies all the time and begin to develop as the girls mature into women, or wishing or choosing to be a mother starts the baby off.

Jeff's account of birth is based on the assumption that babies occur spontaneously. I asked him how he would explain about where babies came from to someone who didn't know anything about it.

Jeff: I'd tell them that how you get a baby is: They come out of your tummy.

Me: What if they said, "Well, that sounds like a good idea, but I don't think there's a baby in my tummy. How do I get a baby to be in my tummy?"

Jeff: Just live.

Me: What if they live a long, long time and no baby has started to grow. Do they have to do something to make it grow?

Jeff: Just wait a long time. Just wait.

Spontaneous birth has as a companion concept universal parenthood. Childbearing is seen as part of the inexorable process of growing up, and all grown-ups are *ipso facto* parents. Categories or definitions of mommies and daddies are not yet developed. Later children will know that it is the begetting or taking care of children that make a parent. Now "a mommy is a grown-up lady," and "all ladies are mommies." To become a daddy a boy need only "eat vegetables" and "get taller and taller." And if they have no children? No matter. They're still mommies and daddies.

Me: How do mommies get to be mommies?

Jeff: I guess they just grow like mommies.

Me: They grow like mommies, and then they're grown-up women.

Jeff: Right.

Me: Are all grown-up women mommies?

Jeff: Yes.

Me: What if they don't have any children? Are they still mommies?

Jeff: They're just mommies anyway.

Me: What is a mommy?

Jeff: A mommy could talk, a mommy could get angry, a mommy could get happy.

Me: What is a daddy?

Jeff: He does work, and he could talk, and he's alive. He could get mad, like mommies could, but my dad is bigger than my mommy.

Asked to define a mommy or a daddy, these children describe activities or characteristics of their own parents. They cannot yet separate the essential from the coincidental ("a mommy paints"), nor can they abstract from the collection of daddies they know to form a category.

Jenny told me, "I have a baby for you. It's in my stomach. It's coming out Thursday—in five days." It's hard to say how deeply held this belief is. The time of exit, at least, seems fanciful. Tina, hitting her belly during acrobatics, cried out, "Oh, that hurts my baby in my tummy!" Rita, at four and a half, described how there are little babies in little girls.

Me: How do daddies get to he daddies?

Rita: Oh, when the boys... the boys are a baby, and then they grow up to a man. The boys grow up to be a man. And they're grown-ups.

Me: But how do they get to be daddies? There are grownups who aren't daddies, aren't there?

Rita: Grown-ups are daddies or mommies.

Me: What if a grown-up doesn't have any children?

Rita:	That's okay. Then the babies are still in the stomach, and then the babies grow to little girls and big girls.
Me:	So, if somebody doesn't have any children yet, what does that mean?
Rita:	That means the babies are in the stomach. I already have a baby in my stomach.
Me:	You have a baby growing in your stomach now?
Rita:	No, it won't grow 'cause I'm little. When I'm big, then it can grow. You might loose(n) the baby. You have to be very, very careful because the baby may get loose in your stomach.

Like Jenny, Tina, and many other little girls, Rita identified with her mother during her recent pregnancy. She liked to play that she too was about to give birth, walking funny, holding her back as she sat down, making plans for her new baby. The line between play fantasy and reality was not always clear. But her belief in the baby in her own stomach is also based on an intuitive deduction. Like so many children her age who believe that babies "just grow" and that an adult woman who is not yet a mother already has within her the baby she will inevitably parent, Rita sees little girls as having even littler babies within them. Picture the nested hollow wooden Russian Matryoshka dolls: As you open each doll you find a smaller but identical version of the same painted face and costume; only the artist's limits in working with small objects prevent the series from being infinite. This toy appeals to children. It makes their view of the continuity of generations concrete.

Little boys, too, may think that babies have been inside mommies since long ago. "I started to be in my mommy's tummy when she grew up real tall," said Alan, almost five. "They're just there all the time," three-year-old Mitchell told me.

Me:	Does your mommy have a baby in her tummy now?
Mitchell:	No.
Me:	How come?
Mitchell:	Because I saw the baby when he walked upstairs.
Me:	What baby?

Mitchell: Jacob.

Me: Could she have another baby in her tummy?

Mitchell: No.

Me: How come?

Mitchell: Because she just doesn't. She won't have another baby.
             Because two, because one baby is just enough.

For Mitchell, *baby* is not an abstract category including all those children recently or soon to be born. It refers only to the concrete existence of the only baby in his life, his little brother. Tina, not quite three, thinks of her mother's unborn child as Angeline, the only baby she now knows. In their conceptual worlds, identity is not yet fixed, constant, and irreversible. Angeline may be all babies, and Jacob the only baby.

It is not only babies whose identities are arbitrary or transient. Children's own identities and those of their parents are similarly in flux. Penny told me, "I can have my mommy be inside me. My mommy's got a tummy. I grow up and be her, be her mommy, and she grows inside my tummy." Erica, also three, announced to her mother that she and her brother were going to grow up and "be you. Danny will be the daddy and I will be the mommy, and you and Daddy will be Grandma and Grandpa." In listening to her, her mother had the clear sense that she was not just talking about adopting different social roles, but of their all becoming other people. The mechanics of these transformations were explained to me by another three-year-old friend, who told me that she would be my mommy when she "grew up" and I "grew down."

Wishes are not just the stuff from which dreams are made for young children. The heady power of an assumed thought magic leads them to believe that wishing something makes it happen. Despite their very real powerlessness, they tend to see the world as organized around their desires and behavior. To be realistic about their own helplessness would pose a crushing handicap to their developing assertiveness and competence. Their egocentrism is not without dangers, however, for the actual turn of events can be frustrating. If a sister dies, if parents divorce, if a teacher gets sick, children often assume that their own anger or misdeeds are responsible for these calamities.

There is a happier side to the magical omnipotence of young children. When asked to explain how come they have the mommies and daddies they do, they regularly claim to have chosen their parents "Because l like this mommy" or because I wanted to have a daddy and he gets me." Some even insist that if they didn't like this daddy or this mommy, they would "get a different one." "If I didn't love him," said Lisa, "I'd have a different Dad." Luckily, this assumption remains unchallenged. All the children I talked with like and plan to keep the parents they have.

If they think themselves powerful, they know their parents to be even more so. Young children often assume that whatever their parents want to do they do, and whatever they do they want to do. Alan's mommy is his mommy "'cause she wanted to be my mommy," and daddies get to be daddies by wanting to be. Seth's sister started to grow in his mommy's tummy because "my mama wanted her to be in there." Some of this recognition of parental power may come from what they have been told by parents who emphasize choice in family planning. But for the children, the desire and the decision are sufficient to make the plan a reality.

A mommy is a mommy is a mommy. But by any other name, she would be somebody else. It is difficult for young children to comprehend that their teacher may also be a mommy or that their mommy may also be a doctor. What is most important, so important that it overshadows all the other roles she may play, is her relationship to them. Mommies get to be mommies, said Alan, because "they just decided to have that name." Grown-up ladies start to be mommies, according to Sally, "when people call them mommies." And Jim is Leslie's daddy "'cause I wanted to call him 'Daddy.'" By giving somebody else a name or renaming oneself, old identities may be discarded and new ones assumed. It is only through diligent repetition and some maturation that children learn that "names will never harm them." For a long time, names are very powerful, and you are what you are called.

Talking with Children

So, now that you know how a child at Level One is likely to think, what can you do with this information? In the "Talking with Children" sections in Chapters 3 through 8, I will discuss how to use what you have learned about children's thinking about sex and birth at each of the six levels. In general, it is a good idea to talk with a child in language which represents one level above where he now is. In this chapter, we will begin with issues to consider in talking with children not yet firmly at Level One.

When your Level One or pre-Level One child asks, "Where do babies come from?" that is just what he wants to know: where? In what place was this baby before it came here? In answering their questions and introducing the subject of new babies, it is best to begin with the geography of reproduction.

Even very young children can begin to understand that a new baby is growing in Mommy's body, although they will need to be told more than once. Children not quite three have told me that the baby is in Mommy's womb and will come out through her vagina. Still younger, preverbal children will lift Mommy's skirt or smock, expecting to see the baby they have been told is in her belly.

A study done more than two generations ago concluded that it is not until they are nine or ten that children first begin to notice and discuss the mother's distended abdomen during pregnancy. Twenty-five years later, I found that even children of two and three made these observations.

Think of how short preschoolers are and how much time they spend looking up at their mothers. What is remarkable and requires explanation is not that they can and do observe the change in her profile during pregnancy, but that this observation is not universal. To not notice such a dramatic change requires a good reason. Most psychologists have traditionally explained children's failure to notice pregnancy as selective inattention to unwanted information. Because they are jealous of their mother's affection, not wanting to share her with a new arrival, they refuse to recognize what they do not want to admit.

While this kind of denial doubtless occurs, it is not the only or even the most prevalent reason why children fail to recognize the fact of pregnancy. More often they lack the labels and conceptual tools to draw conclusions from their observations. If you cannot add, two and two do not equal four, but only two and another two. Mommy's belly may be no larger than those of Grandma and Uncle Joe, who are overweight, not pregnant. Even when Mommy brings the baby home from the hospital, her untutored toddler has no reason to connect his new sister with Mommy's former girth. He has not yet learned to spin the thread of cause and effect between the two events.

When she was three years old, my friend Ana challenged her nursery-school teacher, Jamie. Jamie had just told the children gathered around her, listening to her account of birth, that babies grow inside their mommies' tummies. "No they don't," countered Ana. Jamie patiently explained again. Ana was pleasant but firm. Finally, three repetitions later, Jamie asked Ana where she thought the baby was before birth. "In the mommy's uterus," she answered.

Ana was defending a vital distinction. It is important to teach children that the baby has a special growing place within the mother's body. Children need to know that this special growing place, called the *womb* or *uterus*, is different from and unconnected to the tummy or stomach. Most of the time, some confusion about the precise location of the baby has no ill effects. Occasionally, however, confusion can generate concern.

Jeanne was happy and excited. A new baby was going to come and live at her house, she told her nursery-school teachers. At school, she would pretend to be pregnant, walking with her belly out and her hands at the small of her back. Then one day, with no warning and no word of explanation, she stopped eating. She refused all food both at home and at school. On the fifth day of her enigmatic fast, her worried mother came to school to talk with her teachers about what was going on.

One of her teachers, Rosemary, sat down with Jeanne in the fantasy corner of the schoolroom. They played and told each other stories, and Rosemary learned why Jeanne refused to eat. In her fantasy, Jeanne had a baby in her tummy, just like Mommy. Were she to eat, all that yukky food would bury her wonderful baby. Rather than dump garbage on the fantasized fetus, she denied herself all nourishment. Rosemary explained to her that the place where the baby was had no passageway to either mouth or stomach, but opened only to the vagina, its only entrance and exit. Jeanne, reassured, accepted food from that time on.

Not all children draw the same conclusions Jeanne did. And, of those who do conjure up the same images, most do not attach the same destructive meaning. Alan, for example, told me how he received nourishment before birth.

Alan: When my mommy ate food, it came to me. Yeah, and it was already crunched up in pieces, so I could eat it.

Me: Is that when you were still inside her?

Alan: Yeah.

Me: How did you eat it?

Alan: Well, I didn't eat the food. I didn't eat the things that you would eat with your teeth. Just swallowed the things that you drink. I couldn't chew.

Alan, like Jeanne, had a picture of the food the mother chews falling down to the baby within her. Unlike Jeanne, he saw this as an ingenious way to feed the growing baby. His tone was one of happy discovery. One important difference lies in his not having fantasies of pregnancy, although many small boys do play at being pregnant. Preschool boys may tell their friends that they want to be mommies when they grow up. They do not yet understand that gender identity is forever.

There is a more general lesson to be learned from the different responses Alan and Jeanne had to their shared misapprehension. It is not the confusion itself but the <u>meaning</u> each child assigns his or her vision of events that determines its emotional consequences. A dog may be a beloved playmate or a dangerous beast. Growing up may be eagerly anticipated as promising competence and freedom or fearfully resisted as bringing only heavy responsibility and deterioration. Another author wrote about a little girl who placed books on her head to stunt her growth. If she did not grow up, she reasoned, she would not die. Her actions and her feelings, like Jeanne's, can be understood only by exploring the private emotional meanings evoked by her intellectual conclusions.

Childish beliefs that babies grow in stomachs seldom lead to such dramatic consequences as Jeanne's fasting. They can produce anxiety about eating, especially when children learn that babies grow from "seeds," so abundant in fruit. Having a bowel movement, whereby one might unwittingly and uncontrollably lose a baby thought to be in the stomach, can also be worrisome to the confused child.

Many parents do not even attempt to teach children that the baby grows in the uterus, not the stomach. For one thing, it's a hard word for many children to pronounce. For another, the tummy may be seen as everything located between the breasts and the genitals. If a mother points to her own body and explains, "The baby grows down here, not up there in the stomach," her child may reply, "Well, that's your tummy too.,'

Parents would do well not to let the matter drop there. As we have seen, this is an important distinction, which may require more explanation. The parent can continue:

Parent: That's what most people call the *tummy*. And when a woman is pregnant, it looks like the tummy is growing big. But the uterus [or womb] is in there, pretty close to the tummy, and that's the thing that's really growing.

The child may have some questions at this point. Further clarification may be needed before continuing.

Parent: Then, when the baby is ready to be born, it is pushed out of the uterus through a tunnel in the mommy. That tunnel is called the *vagina*, and nothing can get in or out of the uterus except through the vagina. It's the only tunnel to the uterus. The mouth has a tunnel to the stomach, but it doesn't have a tunnel to the uterus. The vagina goes from the uterus on one end to the vulva on the other end. And that's where the baby comes out.

It is important to add that the vagina is neither the urethra nor the anal opening, but a passageway in women to the special growing place for babies.

Some of the language I have been using may seem like big words for small children. I believe children need to know and have the right to be told the names for body parts and processes. Their tongues may stumble over some of the trickier sounds, so that *bagina* or *gIna* may substitute for *vagina* for a while, but this is preferable to the "cuteness" of pet names that may hinder communication between children from different families. Even when they choose to use slang, children gain confidence from knowing the "real" words.

Children need to know the anatomical differences between boys and girls. Some of this learning takes place through explorations they conduct on their own, with brothers and sisters, playmates, and in the nursery-school bathroom. It is important that parents supplement their children's "self-help" efforts at sexual enlightenment, giving them names for parts of their own bodies and those of the other sex. Direct instructions by parents about female anatomy is especially useful, since the female sexual parts are more hidden and less handled than testicles and penis. If both sexes know about vulva, clitoris, vagina, and uterus, boys and girls are less likely to see each other as sexual "haves" and "have-nots."

Psychoanalytic theory tells us that both boys and girls attach superior value to having a penis and think of girls as having been damaged because they lack this wonderful organ. Little girls then conclude that little boys are naturally superior. Boys agree, and, having seen that girls have "nothing" where their penises should be, fear that they too will be punished by losing their sex organs. One sometimes gets the impression, in reading Freud, that femininity is a deficiency disease for which there is no cure.

There is considerable potential for increasing self-esteem in girls and reducing devaluation of girls by boys in teaching both about female sexual anatomy. The four-year-old boys who told me that babies don't grow in daddies because "daddies don't have uteruses (or "tunnels")" don't think of girls as damaged boys but as having different structures for a good reason. Little girls, lacking the breasts which are the most obvious signs of their mothers' sexual identity, can find reassurance in knowing that they already have a uterus and a vagina for having babies and a clitoris and a vagina for sexual pleasure.

Talking about where babies are before birth provides an excellent opportunity to teach about sexual differences, although this information can be introduced on other occasions as well. A child's "Where do babies come from?" is an obvious time to begin to talk about sex and birth. Helping to diaper a baby or bathing with a sister, brother, or playmate may be other times when a child is inclined to talk about sex differences and reproduction.

Often children don't ask about the origin of babies before they need to know. When do they need to know? Either when all the other kids know or when parents are expecting a new baby, whichever comes first. Children may feel ashamed of their ignorance when talked down to by knowing playmates. More important, they need information which will help them out as they anticipate the changes in their lives that will occur after a sister or brother is born. Will their parents still love them? Will Mother still have time for them? Will Father still pay attention to them, take them for walks, tell them stories? Where has Mommy gone when she's away for several days? Will she ever come back? Children fear they will be displaced in their parents' affection.

"My mommy doesn't want no babies. She always wants to take care of me, to have me," Daria told me. Why does Mommy want a new baby when she already has me? They wonder and worry about the intruder who will disrupt the world as they know it. Where did he come from? Why is she here? How will life he different?

Judy was three years old when her sister was born. Immediately after the birth, she made the rounds of the relatives. Starting with her mother, she asked, "Are you still my mommy?" She asked each family member in turn, "Are you still my daddy?" "Are you still my auntie?" etc. Like all children, Judy thought of the new baby as replacing the old one. She needed to be reassured that her mother can be both the baby's mommy and her mommy too, that Daddy has love and care enough for two children, and that she is still a valued member of the family and not a displaced person.

Children need to be able to share their concerns about pregnancy. They need reassurance that their fears will not become reality.

We have already seen that they may fear that the baby who inherits their crib will also take possession of all parental affection. They may also worry about Mommy's health and welfare.

Jeff, who was not quite four, was eating lunch with his pregnant mother. "Oh, Mommy, my tummy's very full and your tummy's very full!" he exclaimed. His mother explained that her tummy would get bigger and bigger as the baby grew. Jeff was concerned: "Oh, Mommy, your tummy will break." He feared she would burst, like a balloon blown too large. He needed to know that her skin and muscles could stretch as big as the baby.

Later, his mother pointed out the baby's movement to him: "Feel the baby kicking." Jeff, trained to be a peaceable child, didn't think that was right. "It's bad to kick. The baby shouldn't do that." A muscle pain registered on his mother's face, and Jeff demanded, "Did that baby hurt you?' A baby who kicks is violent and hurtful. A less aggressive word, such as *squirming* or *moving*, evokes less painful images.

Even toddlers can be prepared for the arrival of a new baby in the family. Children understand language even before they can use it to express their own thoughts. The younger the child, the less she will understand, but some base will have been laid for the important events to follow. There are several picture books on the market which show families with small children preparing for a birth. Even children too young to speak can look at these pictures, hear the text read to them, and begin to sense that something like that might well happen in their house.

Children love to hear stories about their own beginnings. Hearing about what Mommy and Daddy did to prepare for their birth, where they went and how they planned, helps children feel part of the welcoming team for the new baby. It is easier for them to accept the love and nurturance devoted to the new baby when they themselves feel loved and assured that they received the same care and generated the same excitement. Stories that begin "When you were a baby you used to . . . and I used to . . ." and go on to share a pleasant memory will always find a receptive audience.

When children in his nursery school played "London Bridge," Eddie excitedly announced that he had been in London "when I was in my mommy's womb." London was, therefore, a very special place to him. Lilah told me with pride, "My mom didn't feed me baby food, she fed me only fresh stuff, and I ate it all up, because I loved it." Knowing about themselves as babies, seeing how much they have changed, gives them a sense of their history and continuing identity.

As a guideline for when and how much to tell children, one therapist lists five things children should know by the time they are three or four:

1. They should know the names of the body's sexual parts.

2. They should know the socially shared words for elimination.

3. They should understand the basic fact that babies grow within the mother's body.

4. They should know enough anatomy by direct observation to understand the differences between boys and girls, even if they can't explain how they know.

5. If they want to know and ask about it, they should also know that babies are made by mothers and fathers together.

All this information is within the grasp of the preschool child.

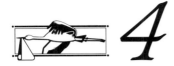

4

The Manufacturers–
Level Two

When a child reaches Level Two, usually between four and eight, he recognizes that an explanation is required by the question how do people get babies? A location where they can be found is not enough to account for the process, and they know it. In trying to figure out the origin of babies, however, they are limited to their own experience of body parts and what each part does, and they also take into consideration the ways they have seen other objects created. A Level Two child knows that babies have not always existed, they must be manufactured. In this way, babies are not unlike other natural phenomena, like mountains, rivers, and storms. For these children, everything in the world has been constructed either by people or by God with magical powers.

Alternatively, children may think that parents are limited to the bodily experiences that children have themselves known. The "digestive fallacy"—the belief that babies get into a woman's body by being swallowed and get out when she moves her bowels—is a generalization from their own body processes. Still egocentric, they assume their own experience is a yardstick of what's possible in the world.

A few of the children at this level assign Father a role in the birth drama, but most of these fit what they have been told to a mechanical process. Father may plant his seed by hand or use his penis to push the seed into its furrow. Magical thinking often broad jumps critical but elusive steps. Perhaps parents need only lie in the same bed together; the sperm may leap from one to the other with no contact necessary, or maybe it rolls across the sheets from father to mother. The physical processes that adults know from personal experience are as fantastic and farfetched to the child as these magical versions are to the grown-up reader.

Imagine a world in which the sun and the moon follow you when you take a walk; when you don't move, neither do they.

• the sea water feels the wind churning waves on its surface.

• when the moon disappears from view it has perhaps gone to see the rain in the clouds, or perhaps it sought shelter from the cold of the night.

• fish know they are called fish; cows and pigs and grasshoppers all know their names.

• clouds are made from chimney smoke from your fireplace and those of your neighbors.

• people cut up the moon so it should look prettier; first full, then waxing and waning into crescents and halves.

• the sun is a ball of fire lit by God, who then threw away the match.

• the clouds are God's breath on cold mornings.

• God is a person who works for children.

For you, this is a world created by a playful imagination. For your children at Level Two, this world may be the only world there is, a world constructed by their developing intelligence, the product of serious problem-solving thought.

There is a story from Jewish folklore of two dull-witted men arguing about when water boils. One maintained it boiled at 100°C. "But," objected the second, "how does it know when it has reached a hundred degrees?"

Piaget uses this folk tale to explain how children regard as living and conscious a large number of objects that for us are inert. Insofar as things show an activity which is consistent and useful to people, those things must possess a psychic life.

Objects which move must then be alive, must know they are moving and want to move where they do. Sun, stars, and moon journey through the universe at their own discretion. Bicycles, motors, and doors feel their motion and can hurt or help you independent of what you do with them.

A child might then replace a half-buried stone dislodged by her foot so that it doesn't suffer from being moved. Considerate of their feelings, she brings home several pebbles or flowers so that they can have company and not be lonely. Perhaps she moves stones from one side of the path to the other, so they won't always have to look at the same view. (Sully/Piaget.)

A man recalls a childhood encounter with a window that fell shut suddenly, nearly guillotining him:

"I was fascinated by the window which I had seen moving by itself like a person and even quicker than I could. I was certain it had wanted to do me harm and for a long while I never came near it without experiencing feelings of fear and anger." (Michellet/Piaget.)

We have all seen children get mad at toys and doors for hurting them, slapping back at the objects they see as causing their pain. Even grown-ups have been known to curse and kick unhearing and inanimate things as they trip over tables, bruise themselves on the corners of bed frames, and put money in vending machines which give them nothing in return.

Endowing objects with will and the ability to move about on their own is called *animism*: animating the inert, granting life to the inanimate, and attributing human consciousness and will to things that operate according to other laws of motion.

Children's questions about the world (Who made the sun? Why do we have dreams? Why is grass green? Where is the baby now that Aunt Ellen will have next summer?) see a purpose for all things. Animism locates these purposes in the things themselves. But purpose, even if it were to inhere in everything always, can alternatively be located in the creator of those things. Then the

creator, be it God or mortal, constructs both natural and manufactured objects alike: by artifice. Piaget calls this way of looking at the
world as if it were manufactured like factory goods *artificialism*. For
children beginning to explore the causes of things and events, the
hows and whys behind the whats and wheres, artificialism, like animism, appears to offer solutions. The sun is a ball of fire God tosses
in the sky above San Francisco from behind the East Bay hills; the
men of Chicago dug Lake Michigan so that the local people might
have beaches to visit; and babies are manufactured by people as if
they were automobiles, TV sets, or dolls. A Level Two child knows
that babies have not always existed, they must be built.

Jane, age four, told me, "To get a baby to grow in your tummy,
you just make it first. You put some eyes on it. Put the head on, and
hair, some hair all curls. You make it with head stuff you find in the
store that makes it for you. Well, the mommy and daddy make the
baby and then they put it in the tummy and then it goes quickly
out."

A year earlier, she had asked her mother, "How do you make
babies?" Listening to her mother's long, scientific explanation, she
looked bored, Fascinated by the bellies of pregnant women, she
pointed them out on the street and asked how the babies get out.
While clear about the location of babies before birth and the exit
through which they enter the world, she puzzled about the process:
The baby belongs to its parents, who wish for and arrange its
arrival. It is still the all-powerful parents who must make the baby.
But how? Why, like anything else that is made by people: by getting
all the ingredients and mixing them together, gathering the components and assembling them to construct a finished product. At this
early stage, children seem to feel no difficulty in thinking of things
and beings as, at the same time, living and artificially made. Even
without the "bionic" heroes that further confound the issue.

According to four-year-old Laura, "When people are already
made, they make some other people. They make the bones inside
and blood. They make skin. They make the skin first and then they
make blood and bones. Maybe they just paint the right bones. They
paint the blood, paint the red blood and the blue blood." When asked
how babies start to be in mommies' tummies, she replied, "Maybe

from people. They just put them in the envelope and fold them up and the mommy puts them in her 'gina and they just stay in there." When asked where the babies were before they were in the envelope, she answered, "They buy them at the store."

Similarly, Tom, a four-year-old boy, suggested that a woman who wants a baby should "maybe get a body . . . at the store"; she could then "put it all together" with "tools" to "produce a baby." Although his mother reported that he had received no religious training, Tom attributed a major role in the theater of creation to God. According to Tom, God makes mommies and daddies "with a little seed": "He puts it down . . . on the table . . . then it grows bigger. The people grow together. He makes them eat the seed, then they grow to be people. Then they stand up and go some place else, where they could live. The seed makes them into people. Before, they were skeletons. At God's place."

Clearly, making mommies and daddies is harder than making babies. A woman who knows the best places to shop and has minimal mechanical skills can assemble a baby. But to create anything as complicated as an adult requires supernatural powers.

These children seem undeterred by the fact that they've never seen a baby factory or a rack of diapered infants at the local supermarket. When provoked by curiosity or directly questioned, they simply make up answers, fitting what they have been told and what they have seen into their way of looking at the world. Because children at this level believe that everything in the world has been made either by a magicianlike God or by people, they assume that babies are created in a similar way.

These children are still egocentric; they can interpret the world only in terms of events or processes they have themselves experienced. Therefore, they often fall into the digestive fallacy and believe that babies are conceived by swallowing and born by elimination. Especially if they believe that the baby grows "in the mother's tummy," children base their theories of the baby's entrance and exit on their knowledge of their own bodies: Anything that is in their tummies must first have entered through their mouths and will eventually leave their bodies when they go to the toilet.

A friend remembers patiently explaining the "facts of life," including intercourse and conception, to her six-year-old son, only to hear him mutter to himself as he walked away from this briefing session, "But I know she really swallows it." Tom talked about God making the skeletons "eat the seed" to become people, and before Laura decided the baby gets into the mommy when "they put them in the 'gina" she suggested that "they just eat them."

Nursing and its role in nourishing the growing baby intrigues young children. Breasts and milk can overshadow the less-witnessed and less-visible aspects of childbearing. When I asked five-year-old Lisa how a woman might get a baby to begin to grow inside her, she replied, "Get some milk in her titties." "How would she do that?" I asked. "Get some milk and just drink it." Tom, when asked the same question, suggested that the baby "eat the mommy's milk."

For many children, it is her having breasts that enables the mother to grow babies. Daddies don't grow babies. in Lisa's words, "because the daddy doesn't have bigger titties, and the mom does."

To eat is to grow, for young children. They are urged to eat nourishing food so that they will "grow up big and strong . . like Daddy and Mommy." We saw that at Level One children said that people get to be parents by "eating vegetables" and "growing up". If you eat, you will grow, and your size is dependent upon how much you have eaten. Jill explained, "My daddy is bigger than my mommy because he ate too much. If my mommy ate too much, then she's going to be bigger than my daddy." So, at Level Two, the baby must eat to grow and the mother may have to eat something to begin the baby's growth. She must also eat in order to gain the necessary size and strength to be a mother. I asked Lisa how mommies get to be mommies:

Lisa: From God.

Me: When do they start to be mommies?

Lisa: From their mothers. They're babies, then they're little children, then they grow up to be mothers.

Me: Do they have to do something besides grow up to be a mother?

Lisa: Yeah. Eat a lot of food, and don't get no cavities, and

I guess have fun.

Me: Anything else?

Lisa: Yeah, get a lot of energy.

If the baby begins by its mother's eating, then it may pass through her digestive tract to exit in the toilet, like everything else that passes through the human body. This belief in birth as elimination is not uncommon among young children, based as it is on their knowledge of their own bodies.

"The baby comes out of a place in your fanny," said Sally. Confusion as to where the baby emerges persists even when there has been accurate education. Two five-year-old boys discussed the location from which the baby emerges:

Allan: It comes out somewhere near the vagina, but not really.

Jerry: They come out of their tush (buttocks).

Allan: No, not the tush. It's somewhere near the tush, but not the tush.

It is difficult to be certain about something you have never seen. Even when the mental image is clearer, the child may wonder, as did six-year-old Adam, "You know what's funny? How could something big like a baby come out something small like a vagina?" It seems like magic.

Other ways out may appear more likely. Children often think of the baby as coming out the belly button, the only way it could emerge directly from the "stomach." This curious knob or cranny must have a purpose, a purpose they correctly associate with babies and birth, and it is the only potential opening in the belly itself.

Even children who haven't heard about Cesarean births come to the conclusion that surgery may be the only way to extricate the infant from the abdomen. The baby is so much bigger than the body's natural openings that a new opening must be needed. Four-year-old Carol told me, "They go to the doctor and the doctor cuts your stomach. I know all about babies." Her mother then told her that she had not been cut out. When I later asked her how she had been born, she changed her story. "I fell out," she said, "the baby falls out, right out." "That would be nice," her mother added.

Sometimes the doctor need not resort to such drastic measures. Five-year-old George said, "Maybe one day Mommy had a hole in her stomach and my brother got out when she went to the hospital, and the man sewed her up with some sticky stuff." "The doctor pulls the baby out, from here," said Sam, pointing to the center of his abdomen. "They go to the hospital," explained Alex, talking of mothers. "And they open up their legs, and the doctor takes it out. From here," he said, indicating his crotch. When questioned further, these children seemed to say that however much the events they describe challenge their logic and the evidence of their senses, the power of the doctor explains everything: "The doctor can do those things."

Seldom does their image of birth center around a passive infant moved along the birth canal by the muscular contractions of its mother. Alex talked about the baby "crawling" through the tummy and out between the legs. Sometimes the imagery grows more violent. "I punched my mommy. I was inside her and I punched the things that was around me and all my water came out. I growed in a little egg in there and then I popped out," explained Jerry. Darryl volunteered, "I know how they get out–they have to fight to get out."

Mark's account of birth was more peaceful, but retains the perspective of the active infant: "The baby grows and gets bigger and then pops out. I don't really mean pop, I mean push. It starts pushing, then sort of winds out, sort of relaxes and sinks out."

Carol, at four, was present at a home birth. She described what she saw: "Born means the baby comes out of the stomach. The doctor comes over your house, and he tells you if you want to have your baby today, someday, and they say yes or no. If they say yes, then the doctor will get it out. You have to push really hard and you have to breathe. You have to keep your body down, not your legs. You have to lie down on your bed, and you need a lot of towels. You have to push really hard while someone's holding your legs. That helps the baby come out. And the doctor's helping you. He tries to get your baby out. He gets all his tools to do that. Yeah, he has some funny scissors and some . . . it's if you cut yourself, it doesn't hurt. And so it's really hard to have a baby. There's a daddy, too. He helps the doctor and you get the baby out. He gets some cottons for the baby, so the blood won't come on the bed. But you need something on you after you have the baby. Because all blood is coming out, and you need to stay in bed for a few days. Because when you're getting up that will help not all the blood come out." Following the birth, she and her three-year-old friend, the older sister of the baby whose birth she described, played at giving birth. In their play they reenacted the powerful scene they had witnessed, this time as active participants, mothers birthing their own infants.

Parents who told me their children knew "everything" about how people get babies would be surprised to hear the stories their offspring told me. We have seen how children can become confused in thinking about what mothers do to get babies and how those babies actually are born. Paternity is still more difficult for the child to comprehend. What do men do to contribute to the growth, or at this level the production, of babies?

Most of the children at this level are clear that a daddy doesn't carry the developing infant in his body. And their explanations for why this is so take into account either physiology or social role. According to Karen, daddies don't grow babies because there would be no way out for the fully developed fetus: "Daddies don't have a hole where the babies come out." Their inability to nurse is another often-repeated reason for why males don't become pregnant. Alex, however, based his explanation solely on reasons of social role: "Because sometimes they have to work and it might come out when they're working, and they'll have to work with it in the tummy. But when there's a baby in the tummy, they have to go to the doctor right away, see. So they don't grow babies." When I asked him whether dads have something to do with the getting of babies, he replied, "I don't know. I think so." "What?" I asked. "They have to find a witch to tell them to turn them into a girl. If they're a girl, she'll know how to get a baby."

Although the magic is seldom this explicit, many children's explanations of paternity depend on fantastic manipulations beyond the realm of the possible. A child who asked her mother how she got in her belly was told "Well, Dad put you in there." She then assumed that he had opened her mother's body and stuck her in, wrapping a fully formed infant in a maternal cover. She didn't know why she had to stay there for a while, except perhaps so she wouldn't get "chilly cold."

Many of these children were adamant that "you need a man and a woman to make a baby" without having any real clarity about the man's contribution. When I asked four-year-old Allan what the man does, his answer reflected the opacity of the concepts involved: "He has something that's like an X-ray, and he uses the X-ray to look inside himself, to see if he has what he needs inside himself to make a baby with." Somewhere in the mysterious caverns of his body, invisible to the naked eye, some unknown ingredient lingers. Perhaps.

At Level Two, many children puzzle over how the seeds get from point of origin to destination. Even when they have been given the facts, they have trouble creating mental images of what they themselves have not seen. And because the truth may be discomforting—the only analogy children commonly have for penetration is their own experience of "getting a shot"—they may try to account for the transfer of genetic materials in other ways. "The father just lies in bed," Carol told me, "until the mother goes to sleep. And then the sperm comes out and comes in the mother."

Sharon had been told that the daddy puts the seed into the mommy on her egg, that the egg and seed form into one piece and grow into a baby in the mommy's womb until it's big enough to come outside and live. So she knew that an egg and a seed are involved in making babies, but she had not been told about how the seed gets to the egg. When I asked her how people get babies, she replied:

Sharon: From marrying people. They put seeds in their vaginas. The mommies open up their tummy, but sometimes they open up their vaginas. So the daddies, so they can put their eggs in them, and they can put the seeds in them.

Me: Who puts the eggs in them?

Sharon: The daddies do.

Me: Are seeds and eggs the same thing or different things?

Sharon: They're different things. An egg is bigger than a seed. And it has a shell. A seed is something that's round,

	and it's too much small, and it grows people.
Me:	What do the egg and the seed have to do with getting babies?
Sharon:	Well, the egg has to be on the seed. And then it grows a baby.
Me:	Can an egg grow to be a baby without a seed?
Sharon:	No . . . 'cause it has to be a special kind of egg and a special kind of seed. The seed is not a growing seed, but a baby seed, it grows babies. It's in daddies' tummies. Eggs are in mommies. And I have eggs in my tummy.
Me:	If the seed is in the daddy, how does it get on the egg?
Sharon:	When the daddy gets it. I don't know how exactly, 'cause he can't really open up all his tummies. Maybe it rolls out. I think the daddy gets it. He puts his hand in his tummy. Then he puts it on the bottom of the mommy, and the mommy gets the egg out of her tummy, and puts the egg on top of the seed. And then they close their tummies, and the baby is born.

For her, the seed and the egg can come together only by manual means. She expressed some doubts that her version of the story could be accurate ("'cause he can't really open up all his tummies") but her experience provides her with no real alternatives.

Barry had been told that Daddy plants a seed in Mommy that has to grow for a long time: this seed becomes the baby, which is born through a special passageway in Mommy. He told me, "One thing I know, how babies are born, that first of all you, they form from a seed in the uterus. It sort of forms in the shape of a baby. It grows and gets bigger and then pops out. Daddies ask the wife if she wants a baby, and then they get a seed and put it in. He gets the seed somehow when he's born. The daddy plants the seed like a flower, I think, except you don't need dirt. He sticks it in the vagina. I think the baby falls out of the seed, and it just cracks open."

Taking the agricultural metaphor very literally, he described the planting of the seed as something the daddy must do with his hands, "'cause the mommy can't reach back to the uterus, to the vagina. I mean she can't reach her arm back." He then thought about that some more and changed his mind: "No, I think she could, she probably could." This ended the interview about how people get babies, however, for he then said that he would like to look at pictures, for "that will probably be easier than thinking." Having decided that the mommy can reach her arm to her vagina, he could not find a reason for the involvement of the father. He remained the seed donor, but there was no longer a rationale for his active participation.

Although they may describe the seeds and eggs with which parents make babies as "special" and "just for growing babies," these children's images remain concrete. Eggs look like those in the refrigerator, and seeds resemble those sown in the garden, with which they may even be interchangeable. Selma Fraiberg recalls a "certain literal-minded fellow of six who was led into minor delinquency by the hopes engendered in him" by the information that "the daddy plants the seed." "He stole a package of cucumber seeds from the dime store and planted them (package and all) under a telephone pole "so's me and Polly can have a baby next summer."

Even children who have learned that the male's material contribution to the baby is called *sperm* are not at all sure what the word means or what the thing referred to does. Carol knew that "sperm comes in fathers and eggs come in mothers." When I asked her what sperm do, she said, "Sperms? You put them in your mama's body and then you look in the telescope. After the sperm comes in then it touches the eggs where the baby are." She had probably seen the sperm described as so small that they can be seen only under a microscope. Their purpose eluded her.

Ellen believed that the sperm were somehow involved in getting the baby out: "The doctor takes the baby out of my mama's belly with a sperm. The sperms help you come out from the belly. The baby goes through the vagina and goes into the sperm, and the doctor takes it out. The sperms swim and then get in. They have to catch to the egg. They have to swim and then they have to hit the egg. They have to catch the eggs because there's babies in it, in the big belly, and the big people have to go to the big hospital to have a baby. Then the baby comes out and you live with it." Although Ellen did not include sexual intercourse in her description, or even identify the sperm as coming from the father, the role in which she cast the sperm was the same as for Laura, who did both.

Laura told me, "A boy sticks the penis into a girl and then the sperm goes in, the sperm goes into the egg and makes a baby. The sperm goes round the egg. Then it gets big and then the baby comes out." When I asked her to tell me more about the sperm, her account became more confused: "The sperm can make a baby come out. It's like from a frog. It has these [drawing squiggly lines in the air with her fingers] things that can make them swim around the egg. And it has a little head. An egg is a little thing that helps people out. It helps chickens. You can eat chicken eggs and birds' eggs, and babies come out of the birds' eggs." "Is the egg that people babies come from like chicken eggs or is it different?" I asked. "It's different, 'cause it's just round. Chicken eggs are like this," she explained, drawing an oval in the air. "What about the egg and the sperm coming together makes a baby?" I continued. " 'Cause the mother wants to make a baby," she concluded.

Karen, too, saw the father's role as helping to liberate an encapsulated baby already formed in the mother: "Well, the dad gets on top of the mother and puts the penis into the mom's vagina. And then it helps the baby come out. It helps the mom get the baby out." Here it is the penis, not the sperm, that permits the baby to leave the mother's body, perhaps by enlarging the pathway.

A creation myth of the Djanggawul tribe of Australian aborigines takes a similar view of the male role in procreation. Their original ancestors, they believe, were a Brother and Sister. The Brother put his index finger in his pregnant Sister's vagina. Then he pulled it away. At the same time a baby boy came out. Sister was careful to open her legs only a little, for if she spread them, children would have flowed from her, as she kept many people stored away in her uterus.

For four-year-old Janet. the father's role was one of protecting the fragile fetus. When I asked her how a daddy gets to be a daddy, she said, "He fucked and the sperms went in, to save the egg, so it won't get cracked. The sperm goes in to protect the eggs. It swims, I think, just like little fishes. So something bumpy won't crack the eggs." She went on to describe how this happens: "Fuck means get on top of each other. And then the thing grows and grows and grows and grows and then they get pregnant and then it comes out the vagina. The sperm swims in into the penis—and then it, I think it makes a little hole, and then it swims into the vagina. The sperm has a little mouth to dig a hole." For her, the sperm is a small animal; if it has a head, then it must have a mouth, and the ability to burrow its way purposefully to its destination.

Like most of the children at Level Two who described intercourse, Janet was not explicit as to how it occurred, but was very clear that it was for procreation only. "They do it," she told me, "when they want a baby they do it, but when they don't want a baby they don't do it." Getting the penis into the vagina, pushing the sperm out through the penis, and having it burrow into the mother, seems so difficult and complicated that it would be foolish to go to all that trouble when you don't get anything as valuable as a baby in return. Another four-year-old attested to the intricacy of this procedure by guessing that "it must have been Saturday or Sunday to take the time to do it." That the sexual act can be one of love and pleasure is difficult for children to understand. Their own experience cannot correct the frequent impression that penetration may be painful and coitus an aggressive act. Selma Fraiberg tells a story of a six-year-old questioning her mother about the imminent birth of the family's third child: "Katie said, 'Mother, can some mothers and daddies try to have a baby and not get one?' 'That's right,' said her mother. 'Gee, aren't we lucky in our family,' Katie said. 'Every time you and daddy tried we got a baby!'"

Although they may not spontaneously conclude that sexual intercourse is making love, a pleasureful expression of affection and closeness, children do seem able to absorb direct information that this is so. Karen told me, "They would do that if they didn't want a baby and they would do that if they wanted a baby." "Why," I asked, "would they do that if they didn't want a baby?" "Because," she said, "they want to hug each other."

Many of the children insisted that parents had to be married to have a baby, sometimes directly contradicting parents who told them that while marriage may be desirable it is not necessary to be married to have a baby. "I have to get married, so I can get a baby,"

Sharon told me. When I asked her why, she had no answer. Karen, too, insisted that "if you want a baby you have to get married. First you get married and then you go on a honeymoon." When asked what about marrying started the baby, she said, "the part when the father sticks his penis in the vagina. But." she added, "they would do that if they weren't married."

Janet's insistence on marriage was more adamant. "If they get a baby, they have to get married," she told me. "Because that's the way you get milk." "How does getting married give you milk?" I asked. "'Cause then the milk . . . 'cause then the man who put the medicine in won't let you keep your baby. The man who took the baby out." The doctor, who delivers the baby and gives the mother medicine to contract her uterus, enforces social convention by impounding babies whose mothers aren't married. Her concern about social convention is a precursor of the preoccupation with roles and rules that characterizes the next level.

Sometimes children generalize from their own family history to the world at large. Two little girls who didn't remember their mother's first husband remember her second wedding as an important event in their own young lives. They were four and six and a half at the time, and very excited to be part of the ceremony. Later, their mother watched as they played with their Barbie dolls. Each time the Barbie dolls would go out and get two children and then go on to marry. To have a wedding without the children being present would be an act of deprivation, barring them from an important family occasion.

"When they get married" is often given as the answer to questions of how mommies and daddies get to be mommies and daddies. Definitions of what a parent is have become more categorical at this level, and adults are seen as having to do something in order to become parents. A mommy "is a girl that takes care of little children" or "who baby-sits, no, who takes care of you." Mommies get to be mommies, said George, because they "growed and growed and growed, by eating. Then their head grows on and then their eye grows on, and then their other eye gets on, and then their arm gets on, and then their foot gets on." If they then have no children, they are not mommies but "just regular people." Before they can be mothers, explained Noah, "they have to cook, they have to teach school, and they have to learn how to drive a car," all necessary skills for motherhood. When asked how come they had the particular mothers they do most children answered, like Karen, "'Cause she's a mommy and I got borned into her tummy." Tom, however, was more fatalistic: "That's the only one God could find."

Daddies, too, are defined by their relationship to their children. "A daddy is a man who takes care of us," Alex said. "A little boy grows up and he's called a daddy," but only "if he had children, like me and my sister." She has the father she does, said Jane, "because Mommy just wanted him." "All the time daddies grow up and then they be child's daddies," explained Carol. "They just tell the mommies that they want to be their daddies." Her daddy was hers "because I wanted to have a daddy and he gets me." When asked why her mother's new mate was not her daddy instead, she replied, "Well, because I want to have a friend." Because biological paternity is more difficult to understand than maternity, fathers still get to be related by wishes that always come true, even after mothers are seen as assigned, at least most of the time, by necessities of the flesh.

The paternal tie can feel like a tenuous one. I asked Julie, whose parents had recently separated, how her father started to be her father. "He's not any more though," she told me. "He's not my daddy any more, he moved." "He's still your daddy, even if he doesn't live here," I said. "No, he isn't," she insisted, "he's just going to come back home lots of days to stay awhile." If a daddy is someone who takes care of children, then a daddy who doesn't is no daddy at all. When biological paternity is still unknown, or only vaguely understood, fatherhood consists of living with and caring for children.

In asking children about the origin of babies, I elicited some stories about the origin of the human species. "Do you want to know how the first people came here?" Allan asked me. "Sure," I replied. "They just, the monkeys turned into people." "How did that happen?" I asked. "I don't know," he admitted, "but it probably was a surprise for the monkeys. Because" he laughed "when they had eggs, instead of monkeys, people came out."

Laura went even further back into prehistory to account for human origins. I asked her how mommies get to be mommies. "Well," she said, thoroughly confusing me for a while, "it starts out to be a plant, and then it grows and grows and then it comes into a person." "A plant grows to be a person?" I wasn't sure I had heard right. "Yes." "How does that happen?" "I don't know," she answered, "but my mama told me it." Later, when I asked her how daddies get to be daddies, I figured out what her mother had said. "They grow up to be a plant," she repeated, "and then they grow up to be a person." "When were they a plant?" I asked. "I think after the dinosaurs were dead. First there was fire in the sky. Then fire fell down and maked rocks. And then the plants growed. And then the plants started out to be persons." "How?" "The plant must have magic in his body," she said, wide-eyed, marveling at a story so fantastic that it must involve the supernatural.

Alex told me the biblical story of creation. I had asked him how mommies get to be mommies, but he found the question too narrow, using it only as a point of departure: "They're in another mommy's tummy, and they grow. And the first people in the world is Adam and Eve. And they ate an apple that God told them not to eat. And God's the one who made the world. And factories make some things, and men make things. But God made the factories and the men made the things in the factories. And you know what? Adam and Eve were the first people that grew. And they could eat any food in the world, but not this tree, because it had apples. And then, they eat one. And they'll become all naked, and they'll <u>know everything</u>, like God, and they'll know how to build things. And people. And so God told them not to eat it, and they did. And then God got so mad he sent them out of the pretty garden. And before, before every time, God was always on the world. And there was nothing. Just darkness. All around. God was all alone, and he decided something: that he was going to build the world. That's the end of my story."

A true artificialist, Alex saw God as the manufacturer who started it all. A little confused about who makes what, his division of labor between God and man seems to hinge on the size of the products involved. Anything as big as a factory must be made by God Himself, while their contents are within the capacities of mere mortals. Yet when people, through their transgression, know all that God knows, they too can build other people.

Talking with Children

In the previous chapter, we discussed how to talk with the child who does not yet know that babies grow inside their mother's body. This knowledge, like other ideas new to children, may not be absorbed all at once. Images of babies bought in stores or hospitals may linger. The child can be gently led to examine his belief, to evaluate it and exchange it for a more accurate one. Following the strategy of talking with children in language that represents the next level of thinking, in this section we will explore how to use what we know about Level Two, the Manufacturer, to talk with the Level One Geographer.

For example, a child may let you know that she believes that babies are bought in stores.

Parent: I can see how you might think that babies are bought in stores. Most of the new things we get are bought at the store. But people are very special. People don't buy and sell other people. Can you think of another way people might get babies?

Child: You get them at the hospital that gives them to you.

Parent: Mommies come home from the hospital with their new babies. So the hospital is a place where something important happens for the baby. How do you think the hospital gets the babies?

Child: They just have them there. The nurses have them, and the doctors have them.

Parent: The nurses and the doctors help the mommy and daddy get the baby. But where do you think the baby was before it was at the hospital?

Child: In another place.

Parent: Yes, in another place, a very special place just for growing babies. The place is called a uterus, and it's inside the mother's body, right here [pointing]. So, the mother has the baby inside her body when she goes to the hospital, and the nurses and doctors help the baby come out.

We have seen that young children have difficulty understanding how "something big like a baby can come out something small like a vagina." They may ask to see the place where the baby comes out. Seeing mother's vagina will not help them understand what they want to know, and she may handle this situation by simply telling them that there are parts of her body that she prefers not to show them. They can be told that the vagina stretches to allow the baby to pass through. Stretching a rubber band can illustrate the principle.

Once firmly established at Level One, children still believe that babies have always existed. While they may know that babies grow in their mothers' bodies and exit through the vagina, their thinking is in terms of the baby's whereabouts and not its origin. The next step is for them to learn that a baby has a beginning, and that people must take action to start a baby.

While parents would not want to offer the more flamboyant metaphors that characterize the Level Two child's accounts of the construction of babies as a craft, children's own thinking is developing in the direction of people and/or God making everything and everybody in the world. Not wanting to tell children accounts of birth and conception that are untrue, parents would not want to talk of putting bones and blood together with curls and eyes to make a baby. But in speaking of putting sperm and ovum together to make a baby, they use a way the child can understand to present accurate information. Let us say that your child has noticed that a neighbor is pregnant. You have talked together about how the baby is growing inside her body. Now, perhaps, your child turns to you and asks, "Where did Ellen get the baby?" By asking a where question, she indicates that her current views are at Level One.

Speaking in Level Two terms, you might say, "Only people can make other people. To make a baby person, you need two grown-up people a woman and a man, to be the baby's mother and father. The mother and father make the baby from an ovum in the mother's body and a sperm from the father's body."

The question of what language to use is important. We have seen that young children are very literal-minded; each word conjures up an image of a real object. They assimilate what they are told to their own experience of the world.

When they hear the word egg, they visualize chicken eggs in the refrigerator or on their plates. When they hear the word seed, their minds wander to planting time in the garden or eating watermelons or pumpkins. Lonnie Barbach writes of a friend who had learned "at the age of five that babies came from an egg in the Mommy's tummy that Daddy fertilized. For years she carried around the mental image of Daddy shoveling manure on a chicken egg sitting on Mommy's tummy."

Even if they don't fully understand what a sperm or an ovum is (and they won't), there is less chance of confusion when parents talk about sperm and ova than when they attempt to simplify by speaking about seeds and eggs. It is especially tricky to speak of ova, because the Latin rule for forming the plural (one ovum, many ova) is so different from the English. Personally, I think that bad Latin is better for children than thinking that they grow from eggs with shells laid by a bird. Remember three-year-old Alan, who said to his mother, "If Daddy put his egg in you, then I must be a chicken."

If speaking of ova is awkward for you, referring to the ovum as an *egg cell* and not simply as an *egg*, describing how the two differ, will help clear up the confusion.

Because *sperm* and *ovum* are new words, they require explanation. For example: "Sperm and ovum are little things in people that are for making babies. Men's bodies make sperm, and women's bodies make ovums. You need one sperm and one ovum to make a baby." If the child is curious to know more, age is no reason to avoid presenting how sperm and ovum get together.

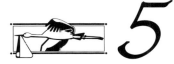

5

The In-Betweens–Level Three

Level Three children range in age from about five to ten. They may know that three major ingredients go into making babies: social relationships such as love and marriage, sexual intercourse, and the union of sperm and ovum. However, their ability to combine these factors into a coherent whole is limited. These children are in a transitional period between the stages of development that Piaget calls *preoperational* and *concrete operational.*

A preoperational child builds mental maps based on her own experiences; she solves problems by intuition. She cannot assign objects to categories. Asked to define an apple, she's likely to say, "It's to eat." As she moves into the next stage, which can happen any time between seven and ten years old, she learns to think systematically and generally about concrete objects. Ask her about an apple now and she'll say, "It's a fruit."

During this transitional period, children are aware that some parts of their explanations don't quite jibe with others. Their accounts of procreation are a mixture of physiology and technology, but they are more insistent than Level Two children that the operations involved be technically possible. Gone are the steps in manufacturing that common experience can readily disprove.

Yet some magical thinking remains. Because ejaculation is as yet outside their experience and fertilization will forever be invisible (except perhaps on Public Television documentaries), these concepts remain elusive, susceptible to infiltration by "supernatural" ideas. They may believe that for sperm and ovum to come together, some manual, medical, or magical intervention is necessary. When the rudiments of sexual intercourse are known, most insist that people would go to all that trouble only when they want a baby.

Because their thinking is still very literal, they are apt to misinterpret metaphors. A sperm described as "looking like" a tadpole may be seen as a separate and complete little animal that can make decisions and move where it wishes. "Planting a seed," a euphemism favored by many parents, may require manually sowing the seed. Love may be as essential an ingredient in baby making as flour is in baking a cake, and marriage may not only be necessary for reproduction, but sufficient. For many children at this level, social conventions are as inexorable as physical laws.

By the time a child is at Level Three, the Age of Reason has begun. Intellectual activity started far earlier, with the toddler's manipulation of objects in play, the questions children rain on their parents, and the fanciful theories they create to explain how everything works and why.

To question, children need only be curious. To invent solutions, they draw on their imaginative ability. It is only when they attempt to verify those solutions, to hold them up to the measure of experience and opinion, that reason is required. Reasoning is the work of controlling and proving hypotheses, thinking to discover the truth rather than for the pure delight of creation. And, true to the developmental insight of Catholicism, children typically begin to reason at about seven.

The need to reason does not arise spontaneously. It is not for ourselves that we work so hard to verify our statements. We do so because other people leave us no choice. Objectivity, as commonly understood, has as its principal criterion the agreement of different

minds. Left to our own devices as individuals, we would immediately believe our own ideas are the sum total of reality.

Experience alone does not always rectify beliefs; things are in
the wrong, not the children who conceived them as different in fancy
than they are in fact. If a mason can build a brick wall and a laborer
dig a ditch, why might men not build mountains and oceans? The
child, who does not work, has little experience with the resistance
of objects. In play, things can be what they wish them to be.

Before they are seven or eight, children have a hard time
telling the difference between physical causality and psychological
or logical motivation. They don't know that their thoughts do not
exist as real events outside their heads. Convinced that adults are
their superiors, they cannot imagine that adults might not understand everything they say and know their thoughts before they voice
them. Even a child who knows that dreams are subjective, so that
she will deny that someone else can touch or see her dreams, may
say that the dreams take place in the room in front of her.

Children's thought is egocentric. Untutored in the art of entering into other people's points of view, they cannot imagine any perspective other than their own. Jimmy may insist, for example, that
while he has a brother named Michael, Michael has no brothers.

The same obstacles that prevent children from adapting themselves to other people's points of view are at work to prevent their
using the evidence of their own senses to construct a coherent world
view. They take their own immediate perceptions as something
absolute. They do not analyze what they perceive, but merely throw
the new in with previously acquired and ill-digested material.
Sometimes they see objects and events not as they really are but
as they would have been imagined if the child had been asked to
describe them before looking at them.

Alert, curious explorers of a fresh, new world, children observe
innumerable details. Having no organizing principle, they have
difficulty in thinking about more than one thing at a time. So they
squander data rather than synthesizing it into packages that can
be stored and retrieved intact.

Children's drawings are a good example of how they depict
reality to themselves. Pictures of tables, trees, and people are not

faithful copies of the objects themselves. But this is not because they are technically unskilled as artists. Instead of looking at an object and trying to reproduce it, children draw only what they already know about things, copying their own mental pictures. A landscape requires grass, trees, and sky; the grass must be on the bottom, the sky on top, and the trees rest flatly on the grass; a house may float in the center of the paper.

It is hard for children before seven or eight years of age to grasp the relations of the whole to its parts. Like "all the king's horses and all the king's men," young children cannot put parts back together again into the wholes they were before being broken down into their elements. But their grab bags of juxtaposed judgments unconnected by any coherent bond does not lead to feelings of chaos or discontinuity. Instead, in the child's mind everything is connected to everything else

Their early judgments do not imply each other but simply follow one upon the other. "And then . . . and then . . . and then," the child's narrative of explanation typically goes, stringing together events without "because" or "although" or "despite," moving from particular to particular without appeal to general propositions. Simplifying and fusing a mixed bag of elements, children retain an unquestioning belief that their condensed versions of reality are the way things are.

Judgments strung together without synthesis act one at a time. Up to age seven or eight, thought teems with contradictions. Boats float "because they're light," so that the strong water holds them up, while in the next sentence a "big boat" is said to float "because it's heavy" and, presumably, strong enough to support itself. Given a complex problem, children shift from one approach to another in a series of attempts. But they cannot reconstruct the route of their meanderings from question to solution if asked how they arrived at their conclusions.

Oblivious to the need for logical justification and unaware of their own thought processes, children see no need to reconcile apparent contradictions. Children may move freely from the egocentric world that has play as its supreme law to the socialized state that demands shared perceptions. Neither of these worlds supplants the other for some time.

But children are none the worse for the dual nature of their reality. They shift comfortably back and forth between belief and play. Each object exists not only as itself but as whatever propelled the child to engage with it, so that a shoebox may remain a shoebox while it serves as a doll's bed. Which is it really? Both.

But these worlds do not remain interchangeable for long. Other people keep insisting that we make sense, that we share their perceptions of objects and events, and when we don't, that we back our assertions with evidence. Social experience gives rise to a desire for system and consistency: judgment changes and reasoning begins.

At about seven or eight, children begin to make comparisons between play and the reality of everyday life. They begin to see the other person's point of view, to realize that if I have a sister my sister must also have a sister, and to put things together according to how they relate to the whole in which they partake. They begin to avoid contradicting themselves, wonder about how what's necessary differs from what's possible, and recognize that chance plays a role in the turn of events. When everything could be justified by referring to anything else, nothing was inexplicable and chance was neither a necessary nor even a sensible concept.

These changes in thinking do not happen all at once. Reasoning is a tricky process. Precausal explanations do not vanish overnight to be replaced by logical, scientific thought. Instead, children's growing awareness that there are points of view other than their own begins an overhaul of their old ideas, which are lined up, taken apart, examined for coherence and communication value, and reassembled. Level Three is a time of conceptual housecleaning, a time of transition during which old thought patterns mingle with the new.

Children at this level explain procreation as a mixture of physiology and technology, but they stick to operations that are technically feasible. Level Three children know that Mommy and Daddy can't open and close their tummies, but they may assume that conception is impossible without marriage. Social roles and social rules have become an important part of the puzzle of reproduction.

Children at this level of understanding may still believe the world of nature is alive; they talk about non-living things and those living things that are not whole creatures as if they possessed will and acted purposefully. Ellen, at seven. said, "The sperm is like a baby frog. It swims into the penis and makes a little hole. It bites a hole with its little mouth and swims into the vagina."

They may also take quite literally their parents' explanations of conception as "planting a seed." The "agricultural fallacy" is still prevalent. Although at this level the seeds don't come in packets from the hardware store, they may still need to be planted by hand. The transfer of the seed from father to mother may take place at a distance, like the cross-pollination of flowers whose pollen is carried from plant to plant by bees and gusts of wind.

Parents no longer have the variety of ingredients available in the marketplace to help them make babies. They are limited to the contents of their own bodies for materials, although they may have to depend on the doctor to supply the critical ingredient. Younger children may believe that "snips and snails and puppy-dog tails" or "sugar and spice and everything nice" are recipes for making boys and girls, but now the metaphor of manufacture includes less-fanciful flourishes. Instead of the freedom of the artist to "get some hair all curls" and "paint the red blood and blue blood," we now see only the concrete addition of parts as the baby grows a head and then a leg and then an arm.

As I've said before, children now may know that three major ingredients go into making babies: social relationships, such as love and marriage; sexual intercourse, and the union of sperm and ovum. However, even those who mention all of these are unable to combine these factors into a coherent whole. During this transitional period children are often aware that their explanations don't quite add up. More knowledgeable about adult criteria for "making sense," they may hesitate to guess about things that confuse them.

Children at this level vary considerably among themselves in the weight given to physiological factors in explaining how it is that babies start to develop inside mothers' bodies. Some confine their discussion to social conventions.

"Well, I first thought, when I was seven," said Isabel at eight, "that all you have to do is get married. And then"—her tone became very dramatic— "all you would have to do is read a book, and then you would have a baby." A year later, she was condescending toward the magic of her former belief, but didn't have much with which to replace it. "I never really got around to how people have babies," she explained, "because I have loads of other things to do." Although she didn't really know what being married had to do with getting babies, she insisted that parents have to be married because "they have to like each other a lot, and they have to share the baby."

Isabel knew that babies start to develop nine months before being born, but she said she did not know what happens nine months prior to birth to start the process of development. Her mother claimed that she had read two books that explicitly described the entire reproductive process. Isabel learned from this that to get a baby you must read a book.

She used to think, just one year before, that "if you didn't want to get married and you wanted a baby, all you had to do is just read a book to yourself, that same book I read, and then you'd have it. I don't know what the book would say." Would it matter? "Well, yes, it would matter. but I don't really know what it would say because I don't go to churches and weddings that much."

To Isabel, knowledge is power. You must only learn the secret of birth to realize its contents, a secret of human creation based on social convention and heavenly covenant. According to her mother, Isabel's sex education by two excellent books "seemed to answer all her questions" since "she hasn't asked since." If, when she asked how people get babies, she was handed a book and told to read it, it was no wonder that she thought books were the single most important factor in the getting of babies.

Even when they can offer no explanation of why marriage is helpful in getting babies, most of these children are orthodox adherents of conventional morality. For them, however, this is no mere social contract, but a law of nature, from which deviation is not only terrible but beyond the realm of possibility. Nine-year-old Larry tried to communicate how topsy-turvy the world would be if marriage were optional to childbearing. He wasn't sure why "you have to be married to be a mother or father," but "if you weren't married and you were called a mother, then it would be sort of weird." The skip-rope rhyme so popular with grade-school girls describes a necessary progression: "First comes love, then comes marriage, then comes [name of skipper] with a baby carriage. How many children will she have? One, two, three ... The better the skipper, the more children she will eventually bear.

Marriage may be seen as sufficient as well as necessary for getting babies. An older child remembered that every time she asked about babies, the response was always "Well, God gets you the baby when you're married." "I thought it was so neat," she recalled, "that God knew that people were married. I thought that it was so neat, like someone could have a baby right after she was married almost, and I decided that was so neat. She must be really chosen, and God decided to give her a baby really quickly after she was married. And then when I found out that the man played a part in it, I wanted to punch the people out, because they took the magic out of it, the magic that God blessed you with this nice baby."

There may be material as well as social and spiritual reasons for marriage. For seven-year-old Karl, marriage was the way to obtain the all-important seed which develops into a baby inside the mother. Fathers get to be fathers when "they and the woman marry," he said. "And then sometimes they get a baby. No, if they marry, then they usually do get a baby. Marrying gives you the seed."

It is vital to remember here that all of the children I spoke with in the original study were either born to parents who were married at the time of their birth, even if they later separated, or were the very young children of mothers who married very early in their children's lives. The idea that marriage is a prerequisite to having babies, carried to the extreme of being a biological necessity, is their own version of what they have been told or a generalization from their own experience. More recent interviews with children who live with never married mothers, who come from communities in which such families are common, or who were born to single birthmothers and then adopted, do not weigh marriage so heavily in their explanations; sometimes they omit it entirely. But they, too, predictably confuse social with physical elements in their stories of how people get babies. For example, they might assume that conception cannot occur without love or that the only way to become a father is to be married to a baby's mother.

Children are now more aware of parents', teachers', and friends' attitudes about sexual topics. Unlike their younger brothers and sisters, who typically answer freely and unselfconsciously, they may show considerable embarrassment and even refuse to answer.

It is difficult to know just what seven-year-old Marie thinks about how the baby starts to develop. When I asked her how the baby comes out of the mother, she smiled and explained her smiling by saying "'cause it's nasty sort of. Well, it's not nasty but its hard to tell you." When asked to advise the hypothetical cave-dwellers about how to get a baby, she said, "I would tell them to 'do it' with a man, and then you'd get one. It's hard to tell you what 'do it' means. I don't really know how you get a baby. I only know that you 'do it,' and I don't know if you eat any medicine or something. I don't really know how to really get a baby because my mother never ever told me about it."

Her mother told me that Marie was taught "sperm/egg physiology" and about "intercourse as a function of procreation and a love relationship," but Marie would describe the baby's growth only in terms of size: "How does it start to grow? Well, it comes out. It just grows a tiny bit when it's in the stomach, and then it gets bigger when it's out. The stomach isn't big enough for someone like you, so it can't grow that big. So that when it gets as big as the stomach can make it, then it comes out."

Her brother Frank, one year older, seems to have absorbed more about the "love relationship" than about the "sperm/ egg physiology." When asked how his dad got to be his father, he said, "Well, he's a doctor and actually he helped with all the stuff, and he mostly did help. (How?) I guess you know. You know I don't like saying it. I have to spell it out to my mommy, because I don't really like saying it."

His considerable embarrassment faded when I suggested he spell to me what he didn't want to say. His tone changed, and he went buoyantly on: "Okay, some people say its p-u-s-s-y, and some people say it's, I don't know the real word for it, but most people say it's f-u-c-k."

What does that mean?

"It's like when people are naked, and they're together, and they just lie together, I guess. Like they're hugging. Some men give hickeys, except my dad don't. They're just together."

What does that have to do with getting babies?

"I don't know. I guess it's like mothers and fathers are related, and their loving each other forms a baby. It's just there's love, and I guess it just forms a baby, like I said before. It comes just by loving and stuff. I guess the love forms the beans, and I guess the beans hatches the egg."

Beans? Yes, beans. To find out what the beans are we have to look at his explanation of how the baby starts to be in its mother's body: "Well, I forgot what those things, ovaries or something. Well, there's like beans which shoot out like, and they come to one of like little eggs or something and they hatch." Perhaps he had seen an illustration of the bean-shaped ovary ejecting an egg and visualized the ovary or "bean" moving toward the ejected egg, helping it to "hatch."

So, love forms beans which hatch eggs. The love between the baby's parents is not just an important part of their relationship but part of the substance of the baby itself, the clay from which it is molded. Fathers get to be fathers "because the lady and the man are married, and he becomes the father because he's related to the baby," He "got related" by getting married. The sexual relationship in marriage starts the baby, but not because the father contributes any actual material to the embryo. Instead, their lovemaking sets in motion the love that will liberate the baby from the egg.

An adult woman I spoke with remembers having beliefs similar to Frank's when she was eight: "I thought love had something to do with it, too. That you fell in love and married. You could only have a baby when you were married, and that wasn't a legal thing, it was a physical thing. And you could only have a baby if you were in love. I remember, I had cousins, and our families were very close. It must have been when I was seven or eight, when Judy's parents were going through a divorce, and she had a three-year-old sister. And I just couldn't understand. I thought, 'Well, gee, they must have been in love three years ago. How come they're not in love any more?'"

According to Diane, the father's contribution is more concrete, but how he participates in procreation remains a mystery. I asked her how babies happen to grow inside mothers.

Diane: That's a pretty hard question to answer. Well, an egg starts to form inside of a mother. And the baby starts to grow inside the egg. Well, the mother and the father, well, like the baby needs to get—if the mother has blue eyes and the father has brown eyes—needs to get the color of its eyes from someone in the family.

Me: Well, if the baby grows from an egg in the mother, how does it get to look like its father, have the same color eyes or hair, or same nose, or something like that?

Diane: Because of the father's genes, I guess. I don't know how they get in the baby. Maybe some special germs.

Germs are contagious. They spread from person to person through close contact: kissing, talking, sharing a glass. Several children mentioned germs in describing how the father's genetic contribution finds its way to the mother. But contagion is no less mysterious than conception. Although conceptually as complex, contagion is something the child has experienced, which makes it a more accessible idea.

The germ theory and other remote control models of fertilization may arise either from ignorance or from generalizing from the pollination of plants. But these theories multiply the dangers they attempt to skirt by increasing the possibility of accidental impregnation. One woman described the distress this kind of confusion can lead to:

"I'd like to share something from when I was a kid. I come from a different environment, Latin America, a different background, and sex was a taboo subject. I remember believing for a long time that babies could come from sitting in a place where a boy had sat. And I would not sit, in a bus or anyplace, anyplace where a boy was sitting. And then that changed to babies come when you kiss a guy. I must have been eight, maybe nine then. And then I was kissed by a boy, and I was completely frightened, crying about it, screaming about it, and not telling anybody. But crying and crying and sure I was going to have a baby."

Getting babies is a medical enterprise in our culture. Babies come from hospitals. They are delivered by doctors (who used to bring them to your home in their little black bags). Even the fact of pregnancy is typically announced following a visit to a doctor. Small wonder that children borrow concepts like germs and contagion from their own medical experience to explain other, less familiar medical manipulations.

The doctor is a prominent figure in children's accounts of reproduction and birth. According to Alice, you need three people, from beginning to end, to make a baby: a mother, a father, and a doctor. She told me, "Well, you have to have a man and a woman. And then you have to have a seed, and stuff from the man, and a doctor and a bed. Then they lie down and the stuff goes into the mother. And they have to get the seed and put it in. And then they lie down and get the stuff from the daddy and put it into the mommy. They get the seed from the doctor—or a store, or something like that—I think it's from the doctor, because the doctor has lots of chemicals that help the baby grow." Both the daddy and the doctor must donate materials to make the baby, and the doctor's contribution seems the more central.

Me: How do people get babies?

Alice: From the daddy. He has something that helps the mommy get the baby. Some sort of medicine. I don't know what it's called, but it's in here. (She pointed to her crotch.) Well, it goes in to some sort of part, I think it's the vagina, and just fixes up and helps around there, and makes it have a baby.

Me: Can she have a baby if that doesn't happen?

Alice: I'm not sure because my mommy never told me if you really need that stuff from the daddy to make the baby or not. I don't think a baby can grow without that because I think it fixes up some special part in there. Maybe it loosens things so the baby can get out when it's time. And fixes up, you know, things that are in there might not be situated in the right place so it takes them and it moves them and fixes it all up.

Me: Is the baby there before that happens?

Alice: Well, it has to have a seed, and then the baby's inside the teeny-weeny little seed. I don't know where they get the seed, but the doctor puts them in the vagina.

Me: The doctor puts it in the vagina?

Alice: I think . . . or the daddy. I'm not sure, but maybe the daddy. I don't really know where he gets the seed. Maybe from the doctor.

Me: What's the seed?

Alice: Well, it's just a little seed that has to have a little baby inside it. Well, they put it in, and then, see, it's the baby. And then the seed grows to be a baby.

Me: What kind of a situation is needed for the seed to become a baby?

Alice: Well, the man puts his stuff into the mother. And that fixes up some of it. That stuff is not the seed, it's something to help around it.

Me: How come sometimes there's a baby growing inside a woman and sometimes there isn't?

Alice: The reason why sometimes there isn't is because they don't have the seed in. Or the stuff from the man. And there is a baby growing, because the seed is in there, and they do have the stuff from the man.

Me: Do they get a baby every time the man puts that stuff in?

Alice: Well, maybe the doctor puts in some more stuff to situate the baby, so it can grow and grow and you know.

Me: How does the man put the stuff in?

Alice: They lie down and, I don't know if it just squirts out. Maybe the doctor takes it out and puts it in or something. Maybe it just comes out through his penis. Or maybe some other place, 'cause I don't really stare at them all the time. I can't know where everything is. They lie down and they put them together. So in case it just comes out, it goes into the mommy.

Me: Do they do that because they want a baby?

Alice: Yes.

Me: Would they do that if they didn't want a baby?

Alice: No. Well, they really have to want a baby to get one, 'cause it's lots and lots of work. If you just do it for nothing, they think, "Well, this is hard work."

Me: Is the work once the baby is already born or before?

Alice: Well, to get the baby. If I don't want this baby, then why do I do the work to get it?

Me: What's the work?

Alice: Well, getting them together, and getting the seed, and going to the doctor.

The father's "stuff," working like a handyman, "fixes up" and "helps around," "situates" and moves the baby "to the right place," and expedites its exit. The father also loves the baby, and its mother, for he gets to be a father by marrying her. But it is the doctor who plays the starring role here—as the source of the seed which comes with a complete baby inside. The mother and father simply provide the appropriate environment for its development. The physician might also be required to get the "stuff" out of the father and into the mother, and he takes the baby out "from the same place it goes in . . . 'cause the mommy wants it out." He is truly indispensable.

Even children who describe sexual intercourse may still find the process mysterious. Ursula, who is eight, described how the father gives "the stuff" for the baby: "Well, he puts his penis right in the place where the baby comes out, and somehow it comes out of there. It seems like magic sort of, 'cause it just comes out. Sometimes I think the father pushes, maybe." But ejaculation was not the only mystery. She was also hazy about what goes where in sexual coupling. When asked if her father did something else besides marry her mother "to help get (you) born," she replied: "He took the part, not his penis but there's another part, two parts, down here, and he took those and then he put them inside. And then the stuff came out, the shell of it. And that's another thing that helped."

So fathers get to be fathers by donating material from their own bodies which contribute to the formation of their children. According to Ursula, there is no baby until the father gives his part, but she was somewhat vague in describing why his contribution is necessary: "Well, the father puts the shell. I forget what it's called, but he puts something in for the egg. If he didn't, then a baby wouldn't come. Because it needs the stuff that the father gives. It helps it grow. I think that stuff has the food part, maybe, and maybe it helps protect it. I think he gives the shell part, and the shell part I think is the skin."

She derives her image of an egg from seeing eggs in the refrigerator. She makes a subtle and interesting extension of her observation of social roles in describing the part fathers play in making babies. The father's culturally defined role as protector is extended to his genetic contribution. He is seen as furnishing the protective shell, the outer covering of the egg, which is then transformed into skin, the outer covering of the person.

Ursula described the growth of the embryo as a rather concrete assemblage of parts: "The egg gets bigger and bigger. It just grows and grows until it's a baby. And it starts changing. Like it starts to grow on a leg. And it starts to grow on a hand. And arms. And when the arms and legs are completed, then the hands, and fingers. And then the feet and toes." As in the manufacture of factory goods, each part is completed before another is assembled.

Ursula was one of the first children I talked with to mention birth control. Most of the children at this level or preceding levels understood family size as an expression of parents' wishes that needed no technical implementation. Or, in a more fatalistic vein, a mother had as many children as happened to be inside her, usually stipulated as the number of children currently in the child's own family. Ursula, however, was aware that people can make decisions that determine whether or not babies are begun. When asked if a couple will have a baby "every time the father gives his stuff to the mother," Ursula replied, "Well, they have to decide if they want to have a baby. And if they don't then the father can't give it. But the mother takes the pill if they don't want a baby. The pills make it so there won't be any egg down in here. So nothing can make the egg."

While she accurately described how pills work to prevent conception, it is hard to tell from her account why they might be necessary, since the father "can't give his stuff" if they don't want a baby. When I asked her if he might give it anyway, she said, "Even if he gave his stuff, it wouldn't work. But," she added ,"he wouldn't do it."

Carol, a particularly precocious four-year-old, was clear about the essentials: "It takes two grownups to have a child like my sister Penny. And they, well the sperm has to go into the lady to be able to have a baby, 'cause the sperm goes into the egg, and the sperm makes life for the baby." She was a bit evasive at first when asked to describe how the egg and the sperm get together, but she soon went on to describe sexual intercourse, which she called "screwing:" "The man and the woman get together in the bed. The sperm and the egg get together when the woman and the man screw. The man puts his whatever-it's-called in the woman's vagina. And then the sperm can wiggle into the egg, and then the egg hatches or something."

"That's the way I learned, and that's the way that people have their children," she replied to my query about why this joining of man and woman, sperm and egg, was necessary. According to her, this takes place when the egg, which contains a preformed baby, has its growth catalyzed by the sperm: "The sperm has the life in it. The egg is for, like the baby is inside the egg, a little something, a seed or something. And then the sperm goes into the seed or something, and the baby develops. The sperm makes life for the baby. It's just, the sperm is like a little thing. It's a squiggily line, and it has a circle there. Here's the egg. It has to go right into the egg. There's like a little hole in the egg. It goes into there and then the baby dissolves, I mean, what's that word? . . . starts forming. And in a few months the baby should hatch, when the sperm goes into the baby's body. I don't know how the sperm makes life for the baby. Just that the sperm goes in, and then that the baby turns out nice. And that's how I learned it, and that's how I know it, because I've only read it, only looked at a little bit of how, the human body book." Carol continually made reference to this informative book, reconstructing its illustrations with finger drawings in the air.

Despite considerable knowledge, Carol's thinking about family size was somewhat unclear. She could think of two reasons why people don't have babies every time they "screw": Either the baby, for unknown cause, dies inside the mother's body or the sperm fails to gain entrance to the egg. People don't "screw" if they don't want a baby, but their wanting and "screwing" may be to no avail if they have already exceeded their quota. Carol, who thought of the baby as preformed in the egg, needing only to be energized by the life-giving sperm, also saw the mother as housing a fixed number of these baby-containing eggs. She explained why her mother was not then pregnant: "'Cause the lady, when they screw, the lady has the children, as many children as she's going to have, come out of her. Well, not exactly. They don't come out all at the same time, 'cause then they'd be all twins or triples, sixes or something." So she answered only to retract her original reply, substituting nothing in its place. Her picture of menstruation was on the right track but hazy: "All eggs don't grow to be babies. If the sperm doesn't go to the egg, if the person doesn't have a baby, they have permanents. They bleed blood into the toilet when they go to the bathroom, every month. Just because the sperm hasn't touched the egg."

Jason's sole explanation of why intercourse does not inevitably lead to the birth of a baby was that the baby died. Nine years old, he told me: When the man lets out this seed or something, and it goes into the mother, the woman, it develops into a baby. And then it grows into a baby, and then she gets pregnant, and then she goes into the hospital and she has the baby. Not all the time. Sometimes it dies when it's in the stomach. Maybe it didn't develop right. Sometimes they don't get enough food or something. Maybe the heart didn't develop right. Sometimes the baby dies."

Tamara was also nine when I asked her how people get babies, and she went straight to the basics: "Well, the mother and the father, the husband and the wife fuck, and then about nine, yeah, nine months after that she sort of feels it, and she thinks it's coming."

I never assumed that because a child used a word that she must know the adult usage of that word, be it street language or technical terminology. I asked Tamara to define *fuck*. She explained further: "Well, when the penis goes into the vagina. And there's a hole where it should go into. And then, it's like they put a sperm together and it starts, deforming."

Amid the malapropism–*sperm* for *embryo* and *deforming* for *developing*–her concept of the baby's beginnings emerged. Its formation involved genital contact but no exchange or transfer of genetic materials: "That little sperm is the baby. They make it when they add, when the penis goes into the vagina, they make the sperm. I don't know how exactly. I think it's the man who makes the sperm. And the woman helps, I think. Well, she doesn't give her help, but the vagina helps. Because you need two, of course, to get a baby, but you need two, I think actually it is two, to start a sperm. Two people. A man and a woman."

How do they start a sperm?

"Well, I think, but I'm not sure, that the penis goes into the vagina and, well, I think it does something. I was thinking that it might touch something in a body, and then it starts growing a little sperm. Like it might touch some blood, or a blood vein or a bone, well doubtfully a bone, but something around the clitoris. Maybe the sperm comes out from that little thing, near the clitoris. It comes out and it starts. Then I think it might break off, come loose and break off and it stays in that one place, or goes up the stomach."

Despite her considerable knowledge of anatomy, more extensive than that of many of the other children in her age group and most of those older than she, the process was anything but clear. Unlike most of her age mates, she knew that sexual intercourse is for pleasure as well as procreation. When I asked her if people "fuck" if they don't want a baby, she replied, "Well, yeah, one thing like they love each other a lot. And that's known as when you love each other a whole lot. And also some people like doing that." She has told her mother that when she thinks of love she has good feelings in her vagina.

Since she knows that people have sexual contact without reproductive intent, she must also have some notion of why babies do not always result. She knew that there are pills so you won't have a baby, and "also there are pills you can take so you will have a baby." She also had what amounts to a reverse theory of immunity, whereby intercourse becomes effective for reproduction only after an initial exposure: "Well, I think, when you get married, you go on your honeymoon. Well, you don't have to, but you go on a honeymoon, and then you fuck on your honeymoon. Or somewhere around after the honeymoon or something. And that makes it so you've got each other's germs, and then when you do it again you've got a baby. But sometimes you don't do it like for long enough or something like that, and then you don't get a baby. But I know some people that do fuck a lot, and they don't always have babies. Like they've got three children." So, she offered three possible explanations for why each sexual contact does not lead to pregnancy: pills, not having each other's germs yet, or perhaps the would-be parents stop too soon for the penis to "touch," "loosen," or "break off" the "sperm."

Six-year-old Denzel answered my question about how people get babies: "Have sex." After he described sexual intercourse and the meeting of sperm and egg, I asked him if having sex always resulted in a baby. "It doesn't if you put a condom on," he answered. Interviewed in 1994, Denzel is an example of how educational efforts at AIDS prevention in recent years have increased young children's familiarity with the condom as a means of both birth control and disease prevention. Familiar with the word, he is not clear that the condom functions as a contraceptive by providing a physical barrier blocking the union of sperm and ovum. Asked why the condom might prevent pregnancy, he theorized "because it tells the stuff that makes the sperm and the egg." Asked if having sex without a condom will lead to a baby in every instance, he waivered: "I think so, but I'm not sure."

Most of the children at this level explain parenthood as a matter of biology or legality. Mothers are mothers because babies grow inside them. Fathers are fathers because they are married to mothers and, perhaps, are needed to start the baby's development. Tamara's explanation of paternity was more inclusive, taking into account the quality of the relationship between adult and child. She first described fathers as getting to be fathers when "they fuck the woman and they've got a child." But then she realized that her step-father was a real parent to her: "I call my dad <u>Dad</u>. I say 'Hey, Dad, you home?', you know, like that, because he is my dad, although he's not the one who fucked my mom and had me." He "is" her dad because he loves her and takes care of her, and because he forms a parenting team with her mother.

Another eight-year-old took a philosophical tone in talking about the destiny of biology: "Well, we have this mother because we have to have her, because we came out of her. And when we came out of her we have to settle for her to be our mother. But I like her." An existentialist, he chose to affirm what he could not change, asserting his power by embracing his fate.

Talking with Children

Following the strategy of talking with children in language that represents the next level of thinking, in this section we will explore how to use what we know about Level Three In-Between thinking to talk with the Level Two Manufacturer.

Remember that the Level Two child usually believes that babies are manufactured. His questions will center on figuring out how construction occurs. He may have doubts about his own explanations; over time his own experience will lead to increased awareness of the improbability of certain key chapters in his story. Perhaps he clings to outmoded beliefs because he has nothing to put in their stead. As he moves toward testing the reality of his ideas, he is getting ready to weed out the technical impossibilities.

Remember four-year-old Jane, who believed that babies are made from eyes and hair and "head stuff you find in the store that makes it for you"? And Laura, who suggested that people make skin and bones and "paint the red blood and the blue blood"? In talking with these girls, a compliment on their imagination and ingenuity is a good beginning:

"That's an interesting way of looking at things. That's the way you'd make a doll. You would buy a head and some hair and put it all together. But making a real live baby is different from making a doll or a cake or an airplane."

These children can be led to understand that while a factory may have a wide range of components at its disposal, babymakers

Parent: Women and men have special things in their bodies that
            they use to make babies. Women have tiny ovum and
            men have tiny sperm. When an ovum from a woman and
            a sperm from a man join together, they grow into a baby
            inside the woman's body.

Children who still think of eating or elimination when trying to
account for how the sperm or ovum gets into the mother's body and
how the baby gets out will need help in sorting out the various
entrances and exits. Parents may have to remind them that the baby
has a special growing place, with its own separate access route, quite
distinct from all parts of the digestive system.

The child who spoke of the daddy who "puts his hand in his
tummy and gets the seed out," while "the mommy gets the egg out
of her tummy," can be questioned:

Parent: Can you put your hand inside your tummy?
Child: No.
Parent: Then do you think the man and woman can really put
            their hands in their tummies?
Child: I don't know exactly, 'cause he can't really open up all his
            tummies. I don't really know.
Parent: There must be another way. Do you want to know how
            they get the sperm and the ovum together? If the child
            says "No," a parent may reply, "Okay, you let me know
            when you want me to tell you more about it." If the child
            says "Yes," the parent might continue:
Parent: The father's sperm are in his testicles, and they come out
            through his penis. The mother's vagina is a tunnel to
            where her ovum are. So if the father put his penis into
            her vagina, the sperm could go through the tunnel to the
            ovum.

The image of the vagina as a tunnel is an important one. We
have seen that children can conclude that sexual intercourse "helps
the baby come out," or that the sperm must "bite a hole" to get to
the ovum. Unless children know that this passageway for sperm and
baby exists before intercourse, they may create fearsome violent
images of the penis forcefully penetrating the mother's body to cre-

baby exists before intercourse, they may create fearsome violent images of the penis forcefully penetrating the mother's body to create the opening. Gadpaille points out that members of both sexes sometimes have fantasies that their genitals, or the genitals of the other sex, may be mutilating, dangerous weapons. Clarity, simplicity, and thoroughness in describing anatomical differences can help prevent these damaging ideas.

It is also good to introduce the idea that sexual intercourse involves love and pleasure, going beyond the mechanics of reproduction to include sexuality and emotion. Children will not spontaneously believe that sexual intercourse is a pleasurable expression of intimacy and caring. But parents who convey that they enjoy and respect their own sexuality can counterbalance children's tendency to think about sex as aggression or, at best, a necessary medical maneuver that takes a lot of time and bother. If Mommy and Daddy are unashamed and say that sex feels good, the child will have a built-in reminder that, appearances and "dirtytalking" classmates to the contrary, it can't be all bad.

This is the part of sex education that most directly involves questions of value. Parents will likely have deeply felt convictions about when and with whom it is okay to be sexually intimate. One possible way of continuing the discussion is suggested here:

Parent: When a man and a woman love each other, they want to be close to each other in many ways. They like to hug and kiss and touch each other all over. That's called making love. When a man and a woman make love, sometimes the man puts his penis into the woman's vagina. That feels very good to them. And that's how the sperm gets into the woman's body to join with the ovum and make a baby. Sometimes people make love to make a baby, but most of the time they make love because they want to be close and loving and because it feels good.

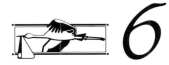

6

The Reporters–
Level Four

Most of the Level Four children I talked
with were between seven and twelve. Although
they may know the physical "facts of life," they
don't understand why sperm and ovum must
unite before new life can begin. Asked to explain
the necessity of fertilization, many children simply describe sexual intercourse and assert flatly
"that's just the way people have their babies"
or "that's the way I learned it."

Called "Reporters" because of their concern
for accuracy, they are reluctant to speculate on
the rationale behind the facts they have accepted
on the strength of the authority of parents,
teachers, or books. Although aware that there
are things they don't understand, they rigorously
exclude theorizing without evidence. At no other
level of reasoning were children so hesitant to
guess when they did not feel certain.

When they do explain why male and female
contributions are necessary to create a baby, the
formation of the embryo resembles a concrete
adding on of parts, rather than following a more
organic pattern of growth. Because they usually
believe that intercourse takes place for the sole
purpose of making babies, they see all babies

as planned and not wanting babies as sufficient for avoiding conception and birth.

They are still engrossed by the social relations of reproduction, attentive to the emotions prospective parents ought to feel for each other, and concerned with how families are started and maintained. Love and nurturance, as well as biological ties, make for parenthood. Love is no longer seen as sufficient to produce a child, but parents must love each other to have a child and must love the child to continue being parents.

By the time the child has reached Level Four, it seems to him as if the world is full of laws. Objects are subject to laws of motion and transformation. A ball of clay rolled into a sausage contains neither more nor less clay than the original ball. Earlier, children claimed that the sausage had more clay because it is longer. Now they see that, although longer, it is not as thick as the ball. They can keep track of the changes in both dimensions and conclude that the amount is the same. They are no longer deceived by an obvious change that temporarily overshadows other changes that balance it out. Perhaps more important, they can mentally reverse and retrace the operation. "If you roll the sausage back into a ball," they explain, "it will be the same as it was before. Since you didn't add any clay or take any away, it has to be the same amount of clay."

Recognizing the equality of two quantities, weights, numbers, or volumes, despite misleading changes in their appearance, is called *conservation*. Conservation is one of what Piaget calls the *concrete operations*. Operations are internalized actions that are coherent, systematic, and reversible. Concrete operations involve real objects that can be seen and touched.

Concrete operations require that we stop focusing only on a limited amount of the information available. Children capable of these mental actions can focus on several aspects of a situation at the same time. They are sensitive to transformations and can reverse the direction of their thinking. They can organize objects into classes and understand which classes are included in more general classes. For example, they can now tell you whether there are more roses or more flowers in a bunch of a dozen flowers, eight of them roses.

For the first time they can coordinate two relations that move in different directions to arrive at the accurate sequence. They can arrange a series of dolls according to height and then give each doll the appropriate size cane from a set of sticks differing in length. They can do this even if the sticks are presented in reverse order from the dolls. What they cannot do is solve a similar but verbal problem: If Joan is taller than Susan and shorter than Ellen, which girl is the tallest of the three? At this level, the child first thinks that Joan and Susan are tall, while Joan and Ellen are short. This line of reasoning leads to the conclusion that Susan is the tallest child, followed by Joan and then Ellen. This solution is the exact opposite of that produced by adult logic about relations.

Children's reasoning that is connected with their actual beliefs, grounded in the direct evidence of their senses, will be logical at this level. Comparisons, relations, inclusion, ordering and measurement of concrete objects are well within their ability.

What they cannot yet do is reason logically about ideas or hypothetical statements based on premises they don't believe. They cannot, for example, tell what is absurd about a sign which reads "Do not read this sign." Either they accept the statement and fail to see what is absurd or they reject the whole statement as silly and fail to grasp the formal absurdity in the situation. Not until eleven or twelve, and the development of what Piaget calls *formal operations*, do children become capable of making deductions about abstract concepts and systematizing their own beliefs. At Level Four, children's thinking is operational but still concrete.

Starting with Level Four, children give primarily physiological explanations of reproduction. They can think logically about objects and people and can consider past and future. They understand the idea of cause and effect. They know that identity lasts a lifetime.

Loath to speculate about things they don't know, children at this level limit their explanations to the facts and nothing but the facts. When their knowledge is incomplete, they refuse to share their guesses or work the problem out further. Although they may know the physical "facts of life," they don't understand why sperm and egg must come together before new life can begin. "That's the way I learned it" or "that's just how people have their babies," they told me by way of explanation. Much of their knowledge is rote repetition of what they have been taught. And respectful of the authority of their sources of information–parents, teachers, and the almighty written word–they feel no need to probe further.

Many of the children at this level first responded to questions about how people get babies with disclaimers: "I don't know much about it," "Well, they just have them," or "I only know one thing." They were aware that there were gaps in their understanding, but, unlike their younger sisters and brothers, they were rigorous in excluding theories they could not back up with evidence.

Only little kids believe in magic. Now they laugh and scoff at their earlier belief in mythical creatures, the elves, gremlins, and Easter bunnies that can't be seen. But neither can they see sperm, ova, the special passageway in women through which the baby exits, or, in most cases in this culture, the mysterious sexual coupling. Trained that seeing is believing, it is no wonder that they are not confident that they can fully explain the invisible events that strain their understanding.

They do know that paternity is a matter of biology as well as social relationships. Most talked about the meeting of male and female cells during sexual contact, although the terms they used to describe the materials involved and the explicitness of their descriptions varied considerably. When parents "mate," "do it," or "make love," according to children who sometimes refuse to clarify what they mean, the "seeds" or "eggs" or "genes" get together and a baby begins.

Why does that have to happen for a baby to start developing? They don't really know and usually refuse to venture a guess.

Fred thought the sperm existed primarily to provide an escort service: "The sperm reaches the eggs. It looses 'em and brings 'em down to the forming place. I think that's right, and it grows until it's ready to take out."

What grows?

"The baby," he said, "the egg," he specified further, indicating that the sperm didn't form part of the developing infant, growing in its special "forming place."

Nine-year-old Fred was uncomfortable, at first, talking about sex. Very aware that many of the words he knew were not acceptable in polite conversation with adults, he kept checking with me about his choice of vocabulary. When I asked him how people get babies, he wavered: "They just get 'em. Well, I know, but I don't know how to put it in words. . . Well, the mother gets pregnant and gets the baby. How should I put it? Well, let's see. Well, then the male and the female mate. Is that a good word? And how shall I say this? Is it okay? Can I say sperm? The sperm reaches the eggs and then just brings them down to some place, loosens them and brings them to some special place."

The place is special, but its location is still a mystery. Other questions remain. "If the tubes are tied in the female, whatever that is, where the eggs are, then they can mate without having a child," Fred explained before going on to tell me that they would not, of course, mate if they didn't want a baby. But wanting a child is not enough. Chance plays a role in the progression of events, and mating does not always result in babies: "Maybe the sperms just doesn't reach the egg right."

Karen, who is eight, explained: "I don't know much about it. Well, I know one thing. The man and the woman get together. And then they put a speck, then the man has his seed and the woman has an egg. They have to come together or else the baby, the egg won't really get hatched very well. The seed makes the egg grow. It's like plants. If you plant a seed, a flower will grow."

Karen's return to the agricultural metaphor is a reminder that children's thought develops in a spiral, not a straight line. They circle back to the same issues but deal with old information at a more sophisticated level.

She knew that sexual intercourse provides a means for the seed and egg to come together. She knew that both are necessary to create new life, but she had no clear idea of why this was so. Nor did she attempt to reason her way to a solution: "Well, see the man and the woman put the, see the man puts his penis into and the lady puts her vagina, and then the man puts his penis in the lady's vagina, and that's how the seed gets to touch the egg. The seed makes the egg grow, and then the egg grows fatter and fatter, and then the baby's inside the uterus. Then the woman who's having the baby gets fatter and fatter. Then after nine months the woman has a baby, and then you go to the hospital and the doctor takes it out."

I probed further, trying to find the rationale for the procedures she had outlined.

Me: Does the seed have to touch the egg for a baby to grow?

Karen: No, if you want to adopt one that's easy to do.

Me: That's another way of getting a baby. But if a mommy and daddy wanted a baby to grow in the uterus, is that the only way to get it started?

Karen: I don't know any other way.

Me: Can a baby grow inside the uterus if that doesn't happen?

Karen: I don't think so.

Me: Every time they do that do they get a baby?

Karen: Well, not if the woman takes birth-control pills, it doesn't happen.

Me: Why do they need the seed to touch the egg for a baby to grow?

Karen: The egg won't hatch.

Me: Can you explain more about what you mean by that?

Karen: 'Cause if the seed doesn't get to meet the egg then it will just break up and nothing will happen. The egg and the seed will just break up. It won't come together like it's supposed to do. The egg won't grow. It just gets split up, and it won't do anything.

Me: What is there about its coming together that makes the baby?

Karen: I don't know.

Me: Can the egg grow into a baby without the seed?

Karen: I don't think so.

Me: Can the seed grow into a baby without the egg?

Karen: I don't know, but I don't think so.

Her facts are essentially accurate. It's unclear, when she talks about the baby or the egg "hatching," whether she thinks that the baby is already in the egg, fully formed and ready to grow if touched by the seed or prepared to disintegrate if things don't go according to schedule. But her image of the egg is still inseparably tied to those in cartons in the supermarket. The Provincial Museum on Vancouver Island has a drawing on the wall of its typical turn-of-the-century bedroom that might well picture Karen's concept of "hatching": It shows a baby crawling out of an eggshell.

According to Karen, babies grow "whenever you want to have a baby," and her mother doesn't have a baby growing in her uterus "'cause she didn't do it." Even children who mention birth-control pills or tying tubes may still maintain that intercourse is only for making babies. Others, who can describe how sperm meets egg, may think that a couple's wishes can determine whether or not a baby will grow.

"Every time people make love," explained twelve-year-old Beth, "they don't always get a baby. 'Cause sometimes they don't want to have a baby. If they want to, they'll have a baby."

How does making love work to make a baby?

"Well, the seeds meet the other seeds, then they make a baby. The seeds from the mother meet the other seeds from the man. And then it forms a baby. Then the baby starts to grow in the mother's stomach, and it keeps growing and growing, and then it comes out. By its head first, so it can breathe. It comes out when the mother's usually in labor. That means when they're in pain, I guess."

I asked her why the seeds have to meet the other seeds for the baby to start. "It just works," she said, "I don't know how."

"The man puts his penis into the lady's vagina," Wilma, who is nine, told me when I asked her how people get babies. "That's all I know." She didn't know what that had to do with getting babies, or so she said, but she doubted that babies could grow if that didn't happen. Nor did she think that a baby would grow every time, "because something goes wrong with the lady's body sometimes, I don't know what." I encouraged her to try to figure out how the babies start to form, but she wasn't interested in pursuing elusive memories. "I sort of learned something that it has to do with their genes in their body but then I forgot the rest," she told me. When

I asked her what genes were, she said she had forgotten that, too, and couldn't or wouldn't guess.

Beverly, who is eight, began by telling me how much her sex education differed from her mother's: "My mother said that her mother told her, when she was real little, that babies come down the chimney by storks. But she doesn't tell me that. She tells me something different. We have this baby book, and it's about how you were born, and all the ways that it's been done. But I haven't actually read the book, so I only know one thing. It comes out of the mother's uterus. I don't know how this works but first there's sort of like this crack in the uterus. And it takes about seven or eight months. And then the baby sort of starts pushing out. And usually there's a doctor with you there, to cut the cord so the baby isn't attached all the time to the mother."

I asked her how the baby starts to be in its mother's uterus.

"The father gives the rest of the egg to the mother. When the man sticks his penis into the vagina."

Why does he have to give the rest of the egg to the mother?

She explained: "Because the mother just has half of it. It's like a egg has two parts. It's just like—we had a big salami, which is whole, and we cut it in half, and we just go like that," she said, bringing her hands together in front of her. "I just thought of the word that happens when two eggs get together. I think it's called the sperm."

What's called the sperm?

"That's when the two eggs get together. The father has one part of the egg and the mother has the other part of the egg. And they have to get together to have a baby."

Again I asked why.

"Well, I think the mother has half of the body, and the father has half of the other body."

"Can you explain some more about that?" I persisted.

"Maybe I could," she said, "but I just can't think of it."

Her version of fertilization is reminiscent of the Alcibiades myth in Plato's *Symposium*. Before birth, according to this myth, we were each part of a joined pair of people. Our task in life is to find our other half in order to recreate the sense of wholeness we dimly remember and long to reexperience. So, for Beverly, the male and female contributions must be concrete and tangible, half a body here and half a body there, like a salami. The fusion of two different cells to form one new entity that is not yet what it will become is too complex a concept to be understood at this level.

Nine-year-old Wanda began by talking about the kind of relationship a couple must have to become parents: "Well, first a man and a woman have to like each other and be with each other a lot. They have to sleep with each other sometimes, and then—do you want the whole everything for the exact stuff, I don't know everything about how it does and things—and then after a long time the woman starts getting a little bit big, starts getting big around here. Then in about six months she has a baby and the baby comes out of here." She pointed first to her abdomen and then to her crotch.

I asked her how the baby starts to grow.

Wanda: From a seed.

Me: Where does the seed come from?

Wanda: From the man and the woman. I think it goes through the man's penis. And it goes into the woman, I don't know where.

Me: Why do they need two seeds, one from the man and one from the woman?

Wanda: To make a boy or a girl. Because otherwise they can't start growing.

Me: How does it start growing?

Wanda: When they meet there's a lot of seeds from the woman going around. The one seed from the man goes and touches, gets one seed from the woman and then they stick together, and then they just start growing.

Me: Tell me more about the seed from the woman. Is it there all the time?

Wanda: It's just there at special times. And some women can't have babies.

Me: Why?

Wanda: When they're about over forty-five, I think then they can't, but I don't know. And some women just can't at any time, but I don't know why.

She has the numbers reversed, giving a lone male seed many female seeds to choose among, and implies that male and female must contribute seeds in order for there to be both girl and boy babies. Perhaps the mother's seed has special duties to perform in making girls, while seeds from the father play the more important part in the formation of boys. We cannot be sure, because she is not.

While children at this level may be unclear about why sperm and ovum must come together to form a new life, they have an intuitive understanding that both father and mother contribute to making children the people they will become. "Who would I be if my mommy had married another man?" they may wonder, knowing that they would not then be themselves. Yet they go on to ask themselves, "Who else could I possibly have been? Because I am me."

A woman I talked with remembered her childhood feeling that she was unwanted because her mother might have preferred another man to her father: "I had a really traumatic experience. I didn't really know until I was in fourth grade that my mother had been married before she was married to my father. And he was my real father, and my brother's real father, but I hadn't known that this other person had existed at all, and when I found out, I was just wiped out. Because I figured that she hadn't really wanted me. It wasn't a divorce. The man died. And I was convinced that she really didn't want me to exist and didn't want to be married to my father. She would have much preferred to be married to the other person. And then I wouldn't have been."

For younger children, mommies are "grown-up ladies" who simply "grew into mommies" regardless of whether they have children. Later, the relationship to children becomes the deciding factor in who is a mommy or daddy, defined as "people who like children" and take care of them. Now both biology and social relationships are taken into account. Children are now aware that the biological fact of birth is accompanied by a set of social expectations about parenting.

When I asked Karen how mothers get to be mothers, she said, "When they have a baby. It just makes that, if you have a baby, you just turn into a mother. It's a special name for the person to have. It's a special name that they call her, and that's how they call them."

"Why do you have this mother?" I asked. Her answer suggests a lottery, in which chance distributes babies among the population of possible mothers: "Because my mother, the people that had me are the only ones that wanted to have me right then, and so then it turned out to be me with them. And so that's why my mother got to be my mother. Seven and a half years ago. My father got to be my father the same way my mother got to be my mother, except he didn't go to the doctor and have me. There's only one person who has me, and that's my mother. But my father's the one who helped hatch me. 'Cause if my mother didn't have the seed, then the egg never would have grown."

Many of the children answered the questions about how people get to be parents by saying simply "when they get married and they have children." Marriage is an even more definitive criterion of parenthood for fathers than for mothers, since they often add that their mothers are "the one that borned me." Fathers get to be fathers when the woman they are married to has a baby. Pressed to explain further, they may add, as did Wanda, "My father got a seed and gave it to my mother, and my mother had a child and that's me, and so he's my father." She was aware that there are other ways as well. When I asked her if that was the way all fathers get to be parents, she replied: "No, not always. They can adopt a baby. Or if they live with a woman, and the woman has a baby, even though he didn't have it, and the woman dies or gives the baby to the man." So love and care, as well as biological ties, can make a person a parent.

Like Beverly, children at this level were more likely than before to form categories to describe parents as "a person who takes care of you," although the group defined by this definition is too inclusive to be accurate. Beverly was also a little confused about the complexities of some family relationships. "They grow up. Then they have to get married, and then they have to have a baby," she said, explaining how mothers get to be mothers. She has the mother she does by virtue of the relationship between her parents. Because she knows from the experience of her friends' parents that marriages do end, she is not sure that parenting relationships do not end with them:

"I have this mother, 'cause my mother liked my father and my father liked my mother. Or else, if my mother and father got divorced I would have had a different mother." "You would?" I asked. "Yes. Well, that would depend on who would, you know, like if my father, he would have to get a new wife. But if my mother took me, she would have to go get a new husband. It would really depend on who would take me."

"Wouldn't your mother always be your mother, even if you didn't live with her?" I asked.

"I guess so," she replied, not entirely convinced. When I asked her how her father got to be her father, she concentrated on the feelings her parents had for each other: "Well, he wouldn't have been my father if, actually if he didn't like my mother, he wouldn't have been my father. If he liked another woman."

"Well, one thing is that he liked your mother. But maybe lots of people liked your mother? Why is he your father?" I asked.

"Once my mother almost married a different guy. And also he used to live in Boston, and my father once liked another woman. But he got to be my father because he just liked my mother better than the other one."

"Did he do anything besides like your mother to get to be your father?"

"I guess they married each other. Well, actually if you want a baby you have to be married. 'Cause the father has one part of the egg, and the mother has the other part of the egg. And they have to get together to have a baby."

So, for her, a loving relationship between the parents was the first prerequisite for having a baby. Then marriage brings the two half eggs together to make one whole baby.

Talking with Children

Knowing that they will soon be Reporters, we can help clear up some confusions for In-Betweens, the children at Level Three, again following the strategy of talking with children in language that represents the next level of thinking. Level Three children already restrict themselves to explanations of reproductive processes that are technically possible. They are busy evaluating many of their former beliefs, reconsidering how lingering ideas from early childhood measure up to their new experience of reality, and rejecting the artificialism and animism of their more obviously precausal theories. Parents now can help clear up misapprehensions, explain why some of their children's beliefs are mistaken, and provide new physiological explanations. Children moving toward Level Four thinking are eager for facts.

Ellen, who believed that the sperm "bites a hole with its little mouth and swims into the vagina," can be led to understand that the sperm does not need to inflict injury on either penis or vagina to arrive at its destination. Like most children her age, she has probably discarded the idea that inanimate objects move of their own free will, acting purposefully as do people; doors, stones, and toys are no longer mistaken for deliberate friends or foes. But mercury, the sun, and objects that move independently may continue to be seen as animate. Sperm, which look like tadpoles and locomote like minnows, are especially difficult to distinguish from complete organisms.

Parent: I know sperm look like tadpoles. And the way they move does look like swimming. But a sperm is not a whole animal. Unlike a fish, it has no mouth to bite with. It can't decide where to go. It just has to move with the semen until it gets near the ovum.

Child: Isn't it alive?

Parent: It is alive, because it's a part of a living creature. Our whole bodies are alive—skin, bones, eyes, stomach everything is made of living cells, tiny bits of living matter. But while all the stuff of which we're made is alive, none of the little bits can think, or move, or behave as a person or an animal can.

Child: Well, then how does it get out of the father and into the mother?

Parent: There's a tube in the father's penis so the sperm can go from the testicles, where they're made, out of his body at the tip of his penis. When the woman and the man are making love, the muscles around his penis pump semen out through his penis into the woman's vagina. That's called ejaculating the semen. Her vagina is like a tunnel, and there's already a hole there so the penis can fit in without having to make a new opening.

Child: It sounds yukky.

Parent: I know. A lot of children think so. It's hard to imagine how good it can feel until you're more grown up. You know how nice it feels when you touch your penis (clitoris and vulva)? Well, that can give you some idea why people like to make love. Sometimes a special feeling called "orgasm" happens, when they feel very excited and after that they feel very relaxed. Both men and women have these special feelings of orgasm, and orgasm is usually the time when men ejaculate.

This is also a good time to help children sort out how feelings and social arrangements for childbearing relate to the physiology of reproduction. Clarity about their parents' values is as important to them as correcting inaccuracies in their ideas.

Values play a vital role in human sexuality. How and with whom to relate sexually is a subject about which everyone seems to have strong feelings. Most parents want to teach their children that sexual feelings are a natural part of human relating, rather than taboo, shameful, dangerous, and requiring either avoidance or repression. At the same time, they would like their children to reserve full sexual expression for a very special relationship, so that it is neither trivialized nor divorced from emotional intimacy.

In talking with children about values, it is important to distinguish among deeply felt principles, social conventions, and physiological processes. While parents may want to teach their children not to engage in sexual intercourse until they feel love for and are loved by, or married to, a partner, no parent who wants to adequately prepare children for eventual sexual maturity will lead them to believe that conception is impossible without either love or marriage.

Frank described conception in the following manner: "I guess it's like mothers and fathers are related, and their loving each other forms a baby. I don't know how it really comes, just by loving and stuff. I guess the love forms the beans, and I guess the beans hatches the egg."

His parents have obviously communicated to him their belief that it is critical that parents have a loving, deep commitment to each other before deciding to have a baby. He has already assimilated this integral part of their value system, and they would probably want to begin by validating that part of his explanation:

Parent: It's really important for a baby that its mother and father love each other and love the baby, so that when the baby is born they can take good care of it. But loving is a feeling and can't start the baby all by itself. A baby is a living creature, and it starts growing from living material. When the mother and father make love, a sperm from the father goes through his penis into the mother's vagina. When the sperm joins with an ovum in the mother, the sperm and the ovum form one new thing, which grows into a baby.

This concept that the sperm and the ovum, once joined, create a new entity that develops into a baby is one that can be introduced to children who talk about each parent contributing "half a body," although it will take some time for them to assimilate this very complex idea.

Marriage, like love, should be differentiated from biological necessity in talking about reproduction. Children can be taught that this valuable social arrangement is important for the baby's welfare without being persuaded that avoiding the wedding ceremony is an effective contraceptive. A parent might say:

Parent: I believe that it's very important that people are married before they have a baby (or before they have sexual intercourse). But it isn't the wedding that gives you the seed. Babies are started when the sperm and the ovum get together during sexual intercourse. People can start a baby without being married, or even without wanting to start a baby. The sperm and the ovum don't know or care whether the people want the baby or can make a good home for the baby. When a sperm and an ovum join, a baby starts to grow. So people have to make sure that they don't let the sperm and the ovum get together until they are ready to take good care of a baby.

This can lead to a discussion of contraception and the parents' values about when and with whom sexual intercourse should occur, and the possible solutions to an untimely pregnancy. It is wise to include the fact that other people may feel differently about standards of sexual behavior, and why you disagree with them. The world abounds with examples of different styles of dealing with sexuality, and it is helpful to children to know where their parents stand and why.

For many children lingering over the remnants of the myth of manufacture, it is the doctor who assumes responsibility for all the elusive, mysterious aspects of making babies. He tells the mother she is going to have a baby and takes it out, and, according to some children, without his intervention the baby might never have begun at all. Some children believe it is the doctor who puts the seed in the mother's vagina; others think he makes the seed from chemicals from his medicine cabinet or that the medicine itself starts the baby. While doctors deserve credit when it is due, this mystification of their importance fosters the illusion that they are omniscient, omnipotent agents of human destiny rather than skilled but fallible health workers whose judgment can be open to question. A parent might say:

Parent: Doctors are very helpful to mothers who are having babies. They can check to see if the baby is growing the way it should and that the mother is taking special care of herself to keep healthy when she is pregnant. They are also very helpful in getting the baby out, especially if there is something unusual happening, like the baby being turned around inside the mother. But people had babies for a long time even before there were doctors. Most of the time, other women came to help the mother when the time came for the baby to come out. Mostly they helped keep things clean and kept the mother company, telling her what had helped them when they had babies.

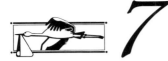

7

The Theoreticians–
Level Five

Children at Level Five are now willing to
speculate about why sperm and ovum must unite
to form new life. Going beyond rote repetition of
the facts they have been taught, they arrive at
theories that echo the history of scientific thinking about embryology. Not quite able to come
up with an explanation of how two things can
become one qualitatively different entity, they
give either sperm or ovum credit for containing
a miniature embryo; the other is relegated to
a supporting role. Either the baby is said to be
really in the ovum, needing the sperm only to cat-
alyze its growth or give it energy, or, alternatively,
it is the sperm that turns into a baby, given the
nourishment and hospitable environment of the
ovum. All see parenthood as a biological and a
social relationship, but most seem to assume that
the physiological aspects of reproduction have
more explanatory value than the social. Children
may begin to give Level Five explanations
between ten and thirteen. It is difficult to set an
upper age limit to this group, since the thinking
of many adults about conception would be classi-
fied at Level Four.

Why am I living?
Why was I born?
Who am I?
Where did I come from?

The intense preoccupation of humankind with the meaning of existence has echoed these questions through the ages. As a species capable of reflecting on our own experience, human beings are denied the unquestioning acceptance of life, birth, and death that marks our brother and sister creatures. Other animals are born, mature, mate, give birth, and die with far greater equanimity than we can muster. Instead, we wonder, question, muse, brood, speculate, and investigate the whys and wherefores of our lives. The more choice we perceive, the greater our need for reason to lead us down the most propitious path. When our actions seem inevitable or unrewarding, we seek some greater purpose that they may be seen to serve.

Prospecting in the hills of life's beginnings and endings, humanity often found the gold of meaning. Mysteries that transcended our ability to see, hear, taste, touch, or smell their secrets, birth and death seemed to promise an answer to the eternal question of the meaning of existence, for birth and death define life by setting its limits.

We saw in Chapter 4 that children's first theories about the world are based on their knowledge of their own bodies, behavior, and thoughts. They personify the sun, the moon, and the wind, attributing human intentions and actions to the world of nature. In this respect, children recapitulate the history of our species. Peoples who preceded us in time also explained the world in animistic terms: the wind as the breath of unseen gods, thunder as the wrath and vengeance of a great spirit, rain or fair weather as gifts from heavenly protectors. Other peoples saw the world as manufactured by an omniscient and omnipotent God, who designed the valleys and mountains, seas and deserts, birds and beasts, all according to plan. Scientific inquiry has revealed, without necessarily challenging the existence of a higher spiritual force in the universe, that the formation of the natural world was not the work of a giant sculptor.

Instead, the creation of the world was a gradual unfolding of physical processes, encompassing a multitude of changes, following natural laws intrinsic to the elements of matter.

The development of children's thinking about many subjects parallels the history of people's beliefs through the ages. Reproduction is no exception. Like young children first discovering how people get babies, earlier peoples first were limited in their knowledge to the fact that babies grow in their mothers' bodies. They, too, wondered where they were before birth, and spun theories of preexistence in other places or previous incarnations. They, too, often believed that the function of sexual intercourse was to open a passageway so that the baby might first enter and then be liberated from its cradle of flesh. Conception remained the great mystery, taking place in head or breast as well as womb, and often depending on the participation of spirits, sun, or rain. There are people alive today who do not yet know about biological paternity.

It was not until 1875 that Oscar Hertwig first discovered that the ovum and sperm each had a nucleus and that the two cells could unite and become one. Two years later, Edouard van Beneden found that the contents of these nuclei were basically similar and that the new cell formed by their fusion then begins to divide into two, four, many cells. In 1879, Walter Fleming witnessed the chromosomes dividing, so that genetic information from each parent could be traced to each cell of the developing child.

Until the 1870s, then, scientists and philosophers throughout history had speculated erroneously about the origin of babies. It was not only people we might label "primitive" who made these errors about the material ingredients that formed the new life, but the wisest and most learned scientists. In pursuing the answers to these age-old questions about the origin of babies, children seem to share many of the beliefs that long characterized the search for an understanding of human beginnings.

A complete summary of the history of embryology would be inappropriate here. What is important for us to explore briefly are two of the leading theories held by investigators for many years because Level Five Theoreticians subscribe to one or the other theory of procreation.

Level Five children believe that the baby is preformed in either sperm or ovum. The embryo is complete unto itself, they believe, and sexual intercourse merely provides the conditions necessary for it to develop. In the history of embryology, *preformation* is used to refer to growth without differentiation. This means that all living creatures were thought to preexist in miniature in the seeds of their parent plants and animals. Preformation theories include Ovism, whereby the embryo is thought to preexist in the ovum, and Animalculism, which claims that the embryo is fully contained in the sperm.

Aristotle expounded at length on Ovist theory. He believed that the material basis for the embryo was provided by the female, while the spiritual component was supplied by the male. According to Aristotle, the semen supplied "form" to the embryo and whatever the female produced supplied the matter fit for shaping; her clay was molded into human form by the sculpting action of the man's semen. His leading hypothesis was that the matter shaped in this way was menstrual blood. Aristotle's theory of conception was based on his belief that the male embodies effectiveness and activity, while the female represents natural existence and passivity, so that her contribution must be material and inert. This theory was elaborated in early Roman times by Pliny, who described how it worked: "The seed of the male, acting as sort of a leaven, causes the menstrual blood to unite and assume a form, and in due time it acquires life and assumes a bodily shape." Sexual intercourse gave "life" to materials already within the female, catalyzing their growth. The father was the provider of spiritual rather than material contributions to his offspring.

From the death of Aristotle, in the fourth century BC., there is little recorded history in the science of embryology until the sixteenth century. Post-Aristotelian Ovists held that all embryos were produced from smaller embryos in the unfertilized eggs. The ovary of an ancestress was said to contain, in miniature, all of her descendants. Before the egg cell was discovered accidentally by Karl Ernst von Baer in the early nineteenth century, Ovists for the past three centuries had thought of the ovum as an oval-shaped body in the uterus. Indeed, ten years after von Baer's discovery a distinguished scientific society awarded a prize for a paper that put forth the belief that the ovum in mammals is first created in the fluid effused from the uterus after intercourse. According to Ovists of that time, the "ovum" merely needed to be "bathed in the spermatic liquor," which would then act upon a preformed embryo in the ovum. Von Baer himself believed that sexual intercourse served to free the ovum from the ovary. To him the ovum was languid and quiescent, requiring the more rompish, energetic sperm to give it life.

Several of the children I interviewed might also be called Ovists. These children seemed to describe the sperm as a catalyst, energizing or giving life to the embryo latent in the egg. Twelve-year-old William was one of them. Asked how people get babies, he replied, "Well, they have intercourse, and then the sperm fertilizes the egg. And then it starts to develop and turns into an embryo. And it starts to grow, and when it's ready, it just comes out."

When asked what fertilization is and how it works to start a baby, he told me, "Fertilize means when the sperm enters the egg. I guess it gives life to it or energy. I guess the egg just has sort of an undeveloped embryo, and when the sperm enters it, it makes it come to life. It gives it energy and things like that."

William had a more detailed, technically accurate concept of other aspects of human reproduction: "Intercourse is when the male inserts his penis into the lady's vagina. And then he has an orgasm, and then that makes the sperm come out. And then that enters into the lady's uterus, and if she has an egg coming down the Fallopian tubes, the sperm fertilizes it and 'comes an embryo."

How the egg "'comes an embryo" is the most complex part of a process that he otherwise understands quite well. He described pregnancy as "when you stop the menstrual cycle and the embryo starts growing, and it turns into a fetus, and keeps just getting bigger." He knew that intercourse did not always eventuate in pregnancy, "because not all the time the lady has an egg in her Fallopian tubes, and when it reaches the uterus and it's not fertilized it just dissolves."

For eleven-year-old Kent, the task of the sperm is to "hatch the egg, so the baby can come out." He guessed that if this were to not occur, "the baby doesn't start to grow, it just stays like this big."

He held his hands about four inches apart. "The sperms make the baby grow."

"Well, they intercourse," he told me in response to my question about how people get babies. "Then the sperm goes to the ovary and it hatches, and the baby grows. Intercourse gets the sperm to the ovary to hatch the egg." He knew that intercourse did not always lead to a new baby: "Well, sometimes it doesn't work. Sometimes you could take pills. And sometimes it just doesn't work, like the sperms don't get all the way through to the ovary."

Kent was one of the few children at this level to comment on the difficulty of talking about sexual matters. "I don't know why it's hard to talk about. I guess it's 'cause it's obscene language. Even though I use it all the time." But talking with the boys in the neighborhood was different from talking with me. "It's because you're a grown-up," he told me, explaining the omissions in his description of procreation and his sporadic laughter. "I don't tell my mother what intercourse means either." "Is it because I'm a grown-up or because I'm a woman?" I pursued the question. "'Cause you're a grown-up. I don't tell my father either."

Like Kent, Kevin was not too clear about how fertilization actually works, but he thought of it as the quickening of a previously static entity: "I don't really quite know what makes it able to work. I guess it just starts it off. I guess it just starts getting a heartbeat or something. I guess it just keeps developing after that." "It" must have already been in existence to get a heartbeat.

Karl's ideas are reminiscent of the Level Three child's shopping list of parts to be collected from mother and father. The hint of concrete assembly of parts is there, but the father's contribution follows Aristotle's thinking about what males have to give to their offspring.

"You said the baby won't grow if the sperm doesn't reach the egg. Why does that have to happen for a baby to grow?" I asked.

"Because the sperm have certain reflexes or something like that that would have to develop in the baby to be born."

"Then what is the egg for?"

"Well, I don't really know for sure, like they could have certain things that have the limbs, or your muscles or something like that. Whatever else the sperm doesn't have."

Later in the interview we returned to the same subject. "Can a baby grow if the egg and the sperm don't meet?"

"No," he expanded on his previous answer, "because the sperm has things like maybe parts of the brain or certain cells that are needed to have a baby or something."

Knowing that both egg and sperm are needed to begin a new life, confused about why this is so and what each might have to offer, he assigned "reflexes" and "parts of the brain" to the sperm. These parts of the nervous system, from which thoughts and dreams emanate and behavior takes its direction, are the material embodiment of the spirituality or life force that the Ovist tradition assigns to the male.

Twelve-year-old Ellen included a more extensive definition of fertilization in telling me how people get babies: "Well, they have sexual intercourse. Then the man, he puts his penis in the lady's vagina and sperm comes out, and they go, if the lady's had her period and if her egg is in her ovary, a sperm will go into her egg, and it will fertilize it, and that becomes a baby. Fertilize means it gives it kind of like ... if a plant didn't have soil or anything, like something it could eat sort of, in a way, it wouldn't really be able to grow. I think that would be the same as with an egg. So fertilize means kind of give it food and things like that."

The idea that the sperm provides nourishment for the egg was unusual, a turnabout of the more common explanation of preformation in the sperm. Perhaps the agricultural metaphor and the list of nutriments on the bottles of plant fertilizer had led to this impression. She was aware that there was some confusion in her story.

"How is it that the baby starts growing when the sperm goes into the egg?" I asked.

"I don't know," she replied. "I guess when it gets in there it just does something to the egg, and it makes it start growing. In some way. I never, in school or anything, they never really explained that in full detail."

"Can the egg grow if no sperm goes in it?"

"I don't think so."

"Can the sperm grow with no egg?"

Her answer epitomized the Ovist solution: "No, that doesn't have the baby. It's the egg that would have the baby in it."

The other side of the preformation coin is Animalculism. In contrast to Ovism, this difficult-to-pronounce theory was based on the ancient belief that genetic parenthood was exclusively a paternal matter. The biblical emphasis on the male seed and the patriarchal line of succession is well known. There is nary a female name in the sequence of "begats" that takes biblical history from the Flood to the story of Abraham. To read Genesis, in which Mizraim begat Ludim... Canaan begat Sidon... Joktan begat Almodad... Shem begat Elam ... and Arphaxad begat Salah, you might think that women had nothing to do with bringing into being each new generation.

In the late seventeenth century, Anton van Leeuwenhoek discovered what he called "spermatic animalcules" by examining semen under a microscope. To many scientists of the two centuries that followed, this seemed *prima facie* evidence that a new baby has its origin in its father's sperm. Leeuwenhoek believed that the ovum served only as food for the sperm, which entered it to grow into a new individual. Unaware of genetic dominance, he was further misled by mating tame white female rabbits with wild gray males. When all the offspring were gray, he took that as proof that the baby bunnies, despite being ushered into the world by their mamas, really came from Papa Rabbit. The common observation that conception does not occur without sexual intercourse and microscopic inspection of the active movements of the sperm were taken as further evidence that the living material for the embryo was furnished exclusively by the father. The disproportion between the head and the body of the unborn or newborn child was also seen as proof that it derived from a sperm, which, they observed, also had a head that seemed to dwarf its tail.

"How do people get babies?" I asked Ollie, who is ten.

Ollie: Intercourse.

Me: What does intercourse have to do with making a baby?

Ollie: Well, the man has a sperm in him that's real tiny and has to go into the lady.

Me: And then what happens to the sperm?

Ollie: It grows into a baby.

It is the sperm that grows into a baby. Ollie made no mention of any material contribution by the mother, who merely incubates the baby. "When the lady has the sperm, the whatever-it-is, the little baby, can just start growing." But the mother must be a careful and considerate incubator. According to Ollie, each instance of intercourse does not lead to a baby, and "If you eat too much, or walk around too much, or if you don't stay down in bed, just stay rested, it will die." It takes considerable effort to provide a hospitable environment for the apparently fragile sperm-child.

In this reproductive scheme, sexual intercourse is necessary in order to transfer the sperm from its point of origin in the father to an environment more conducive to its development in the mother. Twelve-year-old Tessa explained, "I think like the sperm is part of the baby. It goes inside the egg, and maybe the egg is food. Like in chickens, chickens have food. The sperm is something that grows if it gets the right atmosphere or something."

Her description of fertilization gives us a clue as to how her ideas were formed: "The man and the woman have sexual intercourse. The man's sperm goes into the woman's egg and starts a baby. Lots of sperm go and only one gets through, and the egg gets fertilized. Fertilized means—like chickens have lots of eggs, and they don't let them get fertilized because if the chicken's egg got fertilized then it would turn into a baby chick. Instead of just a yolk."

Her knowledge about chickens and her experience of eating their eggs helped to confuse her about people and their eggs. If chicken eggs, left unfertilized, become food, then perhaps the human egg, too, becomes food. If an egg without a sperm does not become a new being, then perhaps it is the sperm itself that grows to be a person when the time and place are suitable.

Eleven-year-old Kathy was more explicit about who does what in becoming parents. When I asked her how fathers get to be fathers, she told me that paternity is predominant in determining who their children are to be: "Well, if they're the man who made love to your mother, then they're your father because you really originally came out of him. And then went into your mother. And your mother, you were born to your mother, but you still have your

father. You were a sperm inside of him there. He has millions of
sperms, and when he let sperm into your mother, only one of them
gets, usually, gets into the egg. And then that one is the one that
gets grown up, and then grows, and then gets born. So that you're
really his daughter or son. 'Cause he was the one that really had
you first."

Kathy explained that the sperm dies if an egg has not been
released, "so that sometimes they have to make love several times
for the sperm to be able to come into the egg." When asked why the
egg must be there for the sperm to develop into a baby, she replied,
"'Cause otherwise the sperm will have nothing to nourish it, or sort
of keep it warm or, you know, able to move or something. It just has
to have the egg to be able to do something—develop. It just dies if it
doesn't have the egg." So the egg is assigned the cultural role usually allocated to women: to provide warmth and nourishment for the
developing fetus. Like mother, like egg.

Robert, at twelve, gave a similar description. When asked what
parents' "going to bed" has to do with getting babies, he answered,
"Well, that's how the... well, the lady has an egg, and the man has
a sperm. And they, sort of he fertilizes the egg, and then the egg
slowly grows, the sperm grows into a baby inside the egg, and
slowly develops, and in nine months it comes out of the lady."

"What does *fertilize* mean?" I asked.

"Well, it means it gets inside the egg, the sperm does, it just
sort of goes in. The egg before the sperm goes in is sort of like...
well, I guess it doesn't have anything in it to grow. It just has food,
and I guess a shell on the outside, or maybe some plastic coating
like a membrane."

"Why does that have to happen for the baby to begin to grow?"

"Well, it's sort of the beginning, the beginning of the baby. It
has to happen, because otherwise the sperm would just die, because
it has no shelter on the outside to keep it alive, no food, nothing.
And then the egg, there's nothing in it to grow, I guess. It has no...
no... no living animal in there. It just has food and the outside. And
he has to put the little thing in there, the man does, and then it starts
to grow. And it just couldn't grow unless that little animal got inside

the egg." So the sperm is a little animal that grows into a bigger animal with the proper care and feeding from the egg.

This quite explicit Animalculist theory of birth, like the Ovist and Animalculist explanations we looked at earlier, echoes scientists' earlier search for the facts of conception. In trying to make sense to themselves in thinking about reproduction, children unknowingly follow the steps of other explorers after scientific truth. Surprisingly, the gender of the children did not seem to influence the theory they adopted, despite the precedence given to one sex or the other by the two theoretical camps. As many girls as boys saw the father as the parent of origin, with the mother providing food and shelter for the baby's growth. And as many boys as girls thought that the baby was really in the egg, with the sperm simply providing the reminder, jolt, or kick in the pants it needed to start growing.

"Well, number one," Robert had told me in beginning his explanation of procreation quoted above, "they probably get married, and they must like each other a lot." Children at this level have begun to see marriage as a social convention that most people follow before having children, rather than as a biological prerequisite for parenthood. A mother gets to be a mother by bearing children. Some consider that she starts to be a mother "when the egg was fertilized in her." Fathers get to be fathers by "sending the sperm into her," or "when the woman has a baby, like his wife or something." Ellen emphasized that paternity is a social role as well as a biological relationship by stating that fathers get to be fathers "by being married to somebody or living with somebody who has a child."

Even though they now know that sexual contact can lead to pregnancy, with or without marriage, they still find it confusing to think about different family arrangements from the ones with which they are familiar. Teri told me that mothers get to be mothers "by marrying and having children." I asked her to elaborate on the connection between the two. "Well, you don't have to be married to have a baby," she replied, "but, um, if. . . I don't know if you can really be a family without being married, or just if you're a family with being married." Although assigning more weight to the physical determinants of reproduction, she was unsure of how to reconcile lessons about marriage as both socially important and physiological-ly extraneous in childbearing. Successful integration of the various factors important in explaining conception and birth seems to require the more sophisticated reasoning of Level Six.

Talking with Children

Up to this point, we have been using the metaphors and thinking style of each level as a basis for talking intelligibly with children who are approaching that level from the level that precedes it. To do so now would be to lead them astray, reinforcing misconceptions rather than helping them to unravel the knots in their thinking.

Instead of talking with Level Four children in the preformist language of Level Five, parents can take advantage of their hunger for concrete information by presenting facts to fill some of the gaps in their knowledge of reproduction. For most children, many processes remain elusive; others may worry about half-digested lessons that irritate their sensitivities as they identify with either parent or fetus. While they both want and need more facts, they are also more aware of their parents' (and society's) attitudes about sexual matters, and may need some reassurance before they can ask questions freely. Embarrassment may persist, for even the most relaxed parents cannot eradicate the influence of the larger cultural milieu, but giggles need not be a barrier to understanding.

Regardless of their level of thinking, girls and boys need to learn about menstruation and seminal emissions <u>before</u> they reach the age at which these may actually happen to <u>them</u>. With the average age of the onset of menstruation, or menarche, steadily declining in Western industrialized countries over the last century, most girls in this country have their first menstrual period when they are between eleven and fourteen years of age, but many begin earlier. For boys, nocturnal emissions, or "wet dreams," typically begin when they are about thirteen or fourteen, but, again, ages vary.

While children need to know about all the bodily changes that will accompany maturation, menstruation and nocturnal emissions are the most abrupt of these changes. Unlike growing taller, changing shape or voice, which may be noticed and commented on as they take place in your own children or their playmates, these less-visible events may occur unheralded. Unless boys know that "wet dreams" are a normal part of growing up, they may worry that they have wet the bed and feel embarrassed about appearing babyish.

Parent: When boys mature, their testes begin to make sperm and their prostate begins to make semen. Semen is a thick, whitish fluid in which the sperm are carried out of the penis. When a man or boy is sexually excited, blood rushes to his penis, so that it gets harder and more sensitive and stands up "erect," which is why that is called *having an erection*. If he continues to feel more excited, if he rubs his penis, semen spurts out of his penis. This is called *ejaculation*, and he will feel an extra-special pleasure that leaves him feeling relaxed and good all over. This is called *orgasm*. Ejaculation or orgasm can happen when he is masturbating or during sexual intercourse or even when he is dreaming about sex. If a boy or man ejaculates when he is sleeping, we call that a "wet dream" or "nocturnal emission," because *nocturnal* means *nighttime* and *emission* means *discharge* or *release*. Men usually ejaculate at the same time as they have an orgasm, while women have the special pleasure of an orgasm without ejaculating.

At the first sign of menstrual blood, uninformed girls may worry that they have hurt themselves. They also need to be prepared about what to do if their first menstrual period begins while they are away from home.

A mother can introduce the subject of menstruation by drawing attention to her purchase of tampons or sanitary napkins. Or a child may ask about these objects seen at home, or repeat stories relayed from other children. In explaining menstruation, diagrams of the female reproductive system can be very useful in showing children the parts of the body involved. After reviewing the reproductive organs, a parent might say:

Parent: Every month, one ovum becomes ripe. This ovum leaves the ovary and travels down the Fallopian tube to the uterus. It travels very slowly. It takes five or six days to travel through the tube, which is only about four inches long. The Fallopian tube is lined with fine, waving cells like hairs that push the ovum through to the uterus. While this is happening, the uterus is getting ready for the ovum to arrive. Do you know how it gets ready?

Child: It bleeds blood.

Parent: In a way. The lining of the uterus gets thick and soft and spongy, because the mother's body directs more blood to the uterus to help form a nesting place in case a baby is started. If a sperm joins with the ovum, they attach to the soft, thick, spongy lining of the uterus, and grow into the beginnings of a baby, called an *embryo*.

Child: What's an embryo?

Parent: That's the name we call the developing baby when it just begins to grow in the uterus. But every ovum doesn't get to form part of an embryo. The ovum is only ripe for a couple of days. If no sperm unites with it, the ovum disintegrates. When this happens, there is no longer a need for the soft lining and the extra blood supply, because no baby is going to be kept comfortable and nourished. So the extra blood and lining pass through the vagina, and the woman wears a tampon or sanitary napkin to absorb the blood. It's not the same as bleeding when you fall and scrape your knee or when you cut yourself. The blood comes out pretty slowly, and it's extra blood, not the blood that is circulating through her body. That's called *menstruation*. A woman has a period, or menstrual period, about once a month, every time an ovum leaves an ovary and there is no sperm to unite with it while its ripe.

I think it is better to speak of the unfertilized ovum, and the also-ran among the sperm in the race to fertilize the ovum, as disintegrating rather than dying. Because children may still mistake either sperm or ovum for a complete new life, saying that either "dies" can elicit funereal images of microscopic moribund babies.

We cannot cover all the questions that may arise for children trying to rethink prior misconceptions and remedy earlier omissions about sex and birth. Some of the more common questions, along with a short reply, follow.

Sexual Intercourse

Child: Janie says the man pees inside the lady to start a baby.

Parent: What do you think?

Child: I don't think pee can help make a baby. But if he puts his penis in her vagina, the pee will go into her.

Parent: I can see how you might think that. You're right that pee can't help make a baby. Urine is a waste product. It's part of what's left over after our bodies use up all of the nourishing parts of the food we eat and drink. Can you think of something else the man might be putting into the woman's vagina when they make love?

Child: Well, he needs to put in sperms, 'cause you need one sperm and one ovum to make a baby. But maybe sometimes he makes a mistake and pees instead.

Parent: He can't make a mistake. Our bodies are made so that those kinds of mistakes don't happen. The penis only lets one kind of liquid through at a time. If semen is passing through the penis, no urine can get in. When a man is having sexual intercourse, only semen can pass through his penis.

Child: Good. I didn't want what Janie said to be true. It sounds awful.

Parent: Do you have any other questions about sexual intercourse?

Child: Well, actually I wonder sometimes . . . grown-ups say they like doing that, but vaginas look real little and penises look too big to fit in. It sounds like it could hurt.

Parent: Do you remember how the baby gets out of the mother's uterus?

Child: Yes, through her vagina. But you said the vagina is just a small opening. I don't see how the baby fits either.

Parent: Most of the time the vagina is a narrow passageway from the uterus to the vulva. But the vagina can stretch large enough for a baby to be pushed through it. After the baby is born it goes back to its usual size.

Child: Well, I guess if the vagina can stretch to fit a baby, it can stretch to fit a penis.

Parent: A baby is much bigger than a penis, so the vagina that can make room for a baby can certainly make room for a penis. Our bodies are wonderfully made to be able to do all the things that people need to do to live and reproduce.

Conception

Child: Aunt Ellen and Uncle Mike say they want to have a baby. Why don't they just have one?

Parent: Not all grown-ups can have a baby as soon as they decide they want one. Sometimes they have to wait a long time for a baby to start to grow.

Child: But you told me the woman's body makes a new ovum every month.

Parent: What else is needed to start a baby?

Child: A sperm. But lots and lots of sperm go into the woman when they sexual intercourse.

Parent: Timing is real important. Both the ovum and the sperm have to be in the Fallopian tube and ripe at the same time. The woman doesn't usually know the exact time that the ovum becomes ripe, and it stays ripe for only forty-eight hours. And even though millions of sperm are ejaculated during sexual intercourse, not all of the sperm are able to get as far as the Fallopian tubes. And sperm only stay active for two to four days. After that, no sperm are available to join with the ovum. So it sometimes takes a long time before the parents can get an active sperm to a ripe ovum, which is the only way a baby can begin to grow.

Pregnancy

Child: How does the baby eat when it's in the uterus?

Parent: How do you think?

Child: Well, I don't think it can eat cereal or bananas or milk with its mouth, like little babies do after they're born. If it opened its mouth, it would just swallow that stuff it floats in. But the baby needs the water to keep it from getting hurt if the mother falls or something.

Parent: That's right. The sac of fluid helps keep the baby comfortable. It always stays the same temperature, no matter what the weather is outside, and it protects the baby by acting like a shock absorber. So how else do you think the baby can get the nourishment and the oxygen it needs?

Child: Maybe through that cord that goes to your belly button?

Parent: Yes, the umbilical cord brings nourishment and oxygen from the bloodstream of the mother to the bloodstream of the baby. That's why the mother has to make sure she eats a lot of good, nourishing food when she's pregnant. She digests the food, and the things the baby needs to grow pass from her blood to the placenta, which is attached to the uterus, and then through the umbilical cord into the baby's blood. So the baby gets all it needs without having to eat. How do you think it gets rid of what it doesn't need?

Child: It can't go to the bathroom.

Parent: No, it can't. But it doesn't urinate or move its bowels when it's in the uterus. Can you think of why it doesn't need to?

Child: The umbilical cord?

Parent: The umbilical cord. After the baby uses all the oxygen and nourishment it needs, the umbilical cord carries the carbon dioxide and waste back into the mother's blood, so that it can be cleansed through her kidneys and eliminated when she goes to the bathroom.

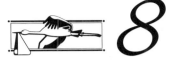

8

Putting It All Together–
Level Six

By Level Six, which may begin as early as eleven or twelve (but may not occur at all), young adolescents have leaped the final hurdle to understand the principle of conception. For the first time they can assimilate the concept that two distinct entities, sperm and ovum, can become one qualitatively different and unique entity, the embryo. Instead of the Level Four Reporter's piecing together of two halves of a body or the Level Five Theoretician's belief that one sex contributes the preformed baby while the other plays merely a supporting role, Level Six requires an appreciation that the genetic materials are transformed in the process of uniting. Now they know that the baby has no material existence before sperm and ovum unite, and that both parents contribute the substance from which it grows.

Although they give exclusively physical explanations of conception and birth, Level Six thinkers are also aware of the moral and social aspects of reproduction. They are able to integrate physiology with emotion, religious teaching, and social convention, taking all into account but differentiating among the role and influence of each. Until this level, the various strands tended to get tangled; now they are woven into one fabric. While they may still make factual errors, these young philosophers' analysis of the process of reproduction is multidimensional and well reasoned. They have begun to use, in Piaget's terms, formal operational thinking.

The path from early questions to clear and accurate solutions is a long one. Along the way, the child runs into mental hurdles that encourage detours. The detours lead back to the obstacles they appeared to avoid. The child is again faced with the same demand for a mental jump, only now the approach is from an angle that makes the leap possible.

We saw that by Level Four the child has discarded the more fantastic, idiosyncratic theories. The Reporters' thinking is no longer precausal, but their "just the facts please" solutions are based on faith in the authority of adults and books. They cannot provide an explanation of the necessity for the facts that they dutifully repeat, and they resist suggestions to think their way through to why the things they describe as being so are so.

At Level Five thought has become more flexible. Children are now willing to imagine the possibilities inherent in a situation and dare to go beyond what they know to be true to explore what might be true. Although their solutions to the question of how people get babies are not completely accurate, their reasoning is more developed and effective than that of the Level Four children, who may make fewer "mistakes." Daring more, they sometimes fall short of the mark, but the exercise improves their capacity to eventually reach their destination. The next step is the realization that the "baby" begins its physical existence only when the genetic materials from both parents have joined and that the traits derived from each are not assembled by the addition of discrete parts. Contrary to popular usage, the child is not a simple composite of "her mother's eyes," "her grandfather's nose," and "her father's temper." More abstract thinking, Piaget's formal operations, may be necessary for Level Six explanations of the origin of babies that reflect children's appreciation of these distinctions.

The last great leap in cognitive development means that people no longer need think only in terms of real objects or concrete events, for they can carry on operations on symbols in their minds.. They

can reason on the basis of verbal propositions, as well as on the
basis of things they can see and touch. They now know, for example, that if Joan is taller than Susan and Joan is shorter than Ellen,
then Ellen is the tallest of the three. To figure this out, the thinker
must be capable of reversing relationships (from "Joan is taller than
Susan" to "Susan is shorter than Joan") and ordering the relationships one at a time or in chains.

For the first time, they can reflect on their own thought. They
can develop theories and test them against reality and can think
about thinking. Confronted with events and attitudes that are not
easily interpreted within their existing ideologies, they see the contradictions as a call to reevaluate both the evidence and their own
beliefs. They begin to be concerned that their beliefs be consistent
and that their actions match their ideas and values. To examine
beliefs in sets for internal inconsistency requires the ability to consider several rules or relationships at once. No longer limited to one-
at-a-time analysis, they can think about events as having many
dimensions, some of which may not be immediately apparent. The
Level Three In-Betweens and Level Four Reporters were confused
about the role of love and marriage in making babies, sometimes
thinking that love was a material ingredient forming part of the
baby's body or that special words said during the marriage ceremony
enabled the newlyweds to become parents. At Level Six, their ability
to analyze the multiple dimensions of an event allows them to consider the emotional and social factors in parenthood without distort-
ing the physiology of reproduction.

No longer is the truth absolute and mechanistic. The context
of an event contributes to its meaning. Earlier a lie was always bad;
now a lie that saves a life may be seen as virtuous. Before, a child
could think that a hostile attack had to be the direct result of his
own immediate action or a reflection that he is bad or unloved; now,
the motive for the assault can be located in events that occurred in
another time and place.

Able to distinguish between their own mental constructions
and the world they know with their senses, formal operational
thinkers are aware that their own experience is only a small sample
of what is logically possible. If you tell a child, "Let's suppose coal

is white," you can expect that child to protest, "But coal is black." Before they are about twelve years of age, children will refuse to consider problems with hypothetical premises that contradict reality, such as: If all winged cats are green, and I have a winged cat, what color is my cat? The younger child cannot disregard the evidence of his senses long enough to recognize and appreciate that the problem creates a self-contained world governed by its own internal rules. If an adolescent is told, "There are three schools, Roosevelt, Kennedy, and Lincoln schools, and three girls, Mary, Sue, and Jane, who go to different schools. Mary goes to the Roosevelt school, and Jane goes to the Kennedy school. Where does Sue go?" she answers, "Lincoln." The eight-year-old might say, however, "Sue goes to the Roosevelt school, because my sister has a friend called Sue and that's the school she goes to." (Kagan.)

The ability to formulate and make deductions from hypotheses that are contrary to fact liberates thinking about relations and classifications from their concrete and intuitive ties. Systematic problem-solving becomes possible only when all the possible solutions are considered and tried. Formal operations allow the thinker to combine propositions and isolate factors in order to confirm or disprove his belief. Piaget devised a task to assess whether children had acquired these mental capacities. Each child was asked to determine what factors determine the speed of movement (or "period") of a pendulum. Several possibilities were considered: length of the pendulum, the amount of weight attached, the height from which it was dropped, and the force with which it was originally set in motion. Concrete operational thinkers varied more than one factor at a time, frequently concluding that weight is a determining factor. Only the formal operational children held other factors constant as they varied one, trying different lengths with the same weight, for example, until they reached the correct solution. (Weight, height of drop, and original impetus are irrelevant. Only the length of the pendulum influences the speed of movement.) Verbal knowledge of science or physics did not help these young experimenters. Their own level of logical functioning was the key to a successful solution.

Level Six answers to the question about the origin of babies seem to require formal operations. Level Five is a transitional period between the concrete operations of Level Four and the more abstract thought possible at Level Six. But formal operations are not universal. While some children become concrete operational as early as five and others as late as nine or ten, everyone eventually does achieve this level of problem-solving. This is not true of formal operations. In a study of lower-middle- and upper-middle-class California residents, formal reasoning was used by 45 percent of the ten-to-fifteen-year-olds, 53 percent of the sixteen-to twenty-year-olds, 65 percent of the twenty-one-to-thirty-year-olds, and 57 percent of the forty-five-to-fifty-year-olds. This means that these mental skills begin to be acquired about puberty, may not be established until adulthood, and for a large proportion are never fully developed. Not simply a matter of tested intelligence, with which is it not systematically related, formal reasoning arises only when maturation, social learning, and life experience permit and require complex, abstract thought.

Recognizing that the embryo begins its biological existence at the moment of conception because both parents contribute genetic materials to its creation is the key to understanding Level Six thinking about reproduction. Children's explanations for the necessity of fertilization ranged from detailed, technical accounts to the vaguer "the fluids have to be together to make the baby" and "the two cells are attracted to each other, meet, and start growing." Regardless of whether the explanations are accurate, what is important is the felt need to seek reasons for the union of sperm and ovum, neither of which is said to contain a preformed baby.

Twelve-year-old Richard began his account of how people get babies by describing sexual intercourse: "Well, the male injects sperm into the female's womb, and an egg forms, and there you have a baby. Well, an egg is fertilized, and it grows into a fetus, which, after nine months of living in the womb, emerges as a baby."

According to Richard, fertilization was necessary to produce a chemical reaction between the sperm and the egg, a reaction that begins the embryo's development. Although he used an agricultural metaphor in defining fertilization, he made a distinction between plants and people: "Let's see, we talked about it in science. Fertilize means to help grow. To start the growth process, like when you fertilize your garden with fertilizer. It's to make it grow."

"Is it the same kind of fertilizing with the egg as with the garden?" I asked.

"It's kind of hard to put. Yeah, it's different. When the egg is fertilized it sort of comes to life. If you want to . . . the chemicals make it come to life. The sperm are injected to where the eggs are, and they just, I guess, coat them. There's some chemical in the sperms that activates another chemical in the egg, which starts the development of the baby."

Mitchell's account was the most scientifically accurate description of conception. At thirteen, his knowledge was considerable. Despite his emphasis on detailed physiological events, he began by underlining the emotional context for making babies: "Well, first of all it's a relationship between two people. And so they decide they want to have a new person in their life. And so they decide that if they are going to have a baby, then they arrange to have intercourse. It takes place sometimes when they feel like they want to have intercourse so they have it. And then it takes a while, nine months is the usual time, but it can be born prematurely or after. So the baby's born, grows up, and so you have a baby and that's about it."

"How is the baby born?" I asked, unprepared for the detail that followed.

"Well, the male has two testicles, and they contain a substance known as semen, which carries the sperm, and it travels through this tube. I forget what the tube is. And it is pumped through the penis into the vagina of the girl, which in this time it goes in and embeds itself. Oh, I'm sorry. The sperm encounters one ovum, and one sperm breaks into the ovum which produces, the sperm makes like a cell, and the cell separates and divides, and so it's dividing, and the ovum goes through a tube and embeds itself in the wall of the, I think it's the fetus of the woman."

Mitchell's substitution of *fetus* for *uterus* underlines an important point. It is the sophistication of the child's reasoning, not simply whether his explanation is correct, that indicates the level of his understanding. Mitchell's verbal error is like the error of an algebra student who understands quadratic equations but makes a mistake in multiplication.

The only child I talked with to mention cell division forming the embryo, Mitchell also outlined the entire maturational process, complete with all the physiological changes experienced by both sexes at puberty. I had asked him how mothers get to be mothers.

"Well, they mature at a certain age. They start maturing basically at the age of—females mature before males, basically they're mature more quick than males. They start maturing at the age of about eleven to thirteen, and they just keep maturing. And they grow much taller, and they perspire, that's when you start perspiring more heavily, when you mature. And you grow hairs on different places, like under the arms and on the vagina and so forth. And that comes from maturing. And the breasts grow slowly, sometimes faster than usual. They grow from about twelve up, and then you stop growing at about . . . oh, I can't remember. But anyhow that's mostly part of it."

The question about how fathers get to be fathers, drew a parallel response: "Well, it's the same process. They mature, more slowly than females. They grow hairs under their arms and on their penis and around there. They perspire more heavily, and, oh yes, acne. You sometimes start getting acne as you mature, as you get older. And as they grow up, if they have intercourse then they produce the baby. And then they start to be a father, and they have to have responsibilities such as taking care of the baby and so forth."

He then went on to discuss various means of preventing conception. When I asked him if people not using contraceptives will have a baby following intercourse, he considered several factors: "After you're old, I mean very, if you're getting very old, you just stop producing, you always produce sperm but the sperm are just too weak, and they don't produce the right way and so nothing happens, you know. Contraceptive devices like vasectomy, which means you can have intercourse without using any other contraceptive like birth-control pills, you know."

"You talked about old people," I said. "What about young ones?"

"Well, it depends on how young they are. You see you start producing sperm sometimes at thirteen, fourteen, fifteen, you just can't tell. See, if you were to have intercourse at thirteen, there are probabilities that you might, something might happen, the sperm might reach the egg, if there are any sperm, sometimes there aren't. And so that makes it very probable because sometimes people produce faster than others. There are just so many different people in the world, maturing differently than others."

Listening to Mitchell, the strength and availability of sperm seemed to be the only factor determining whether conception would occur. I tried to find out if he could think of any other reasons why intercourse without contraception may not lead to fertilization. I asked him, "If people are mature, do they have a baby every time they have intercourse?"

"Well, it depends really, because one time if you have intercourse you might have triplets or quadruplets or something, and you might, well yes, I think so, because you're producing sperm all the time, billions and billions of sperm, you're producing inside you. Producing in cells, like I mean they're cells themselves. So, you know it's probably that every time you have intercourse something might happen. But lots, a third, probably a third of the people use contraceptive devices, and I mean they only have to have intercourse even once or twice, unless you want to have a lot of children, you know. Most people don't have actual intercourse, for the child, more than twice or three times usually. Because they, you know, they can't afford to have that many kids. So they just use contraceptive devices if they want to have intercourse again. They would want to anyway, you know. Sometimes, you know, people do it sometimes just for the pleasure of it. They enjoy it."

Like others of his age, Mitchell knows that sex is not just for making babies. But he is so entranced with the changes going on in his own body, the "billions and billions" of sperm that promise his own future fertility, that he does not shift his focus to consider when and why females are fertile. I was so overwhelmed by the extent of his knowledge, and the comprehensiveness of his replies, that I failed to ask him the critical question: Why does fertilization have to occur to produce a baby?

Tina's reply to that question revealed that she learned about genes at school. Almost twelve when I talked with her, she lacked confidence in her answer, which was well thought out:

"Fertilization? Well, it just, it starts it off, I guess. You know. Well, mixes something. Mixes the genes or, well, puts particles or something into the egg, to make it, you know, fertilized. And so it will, you know, have genes and different kinds of blood and stuff like that, I guess. Because if it didn't, it would be more like the mother, I guess. Genes are the things from the father and the mother, you know, and they put a little bit of each into the baby, so the baby turns out to be a little bit like the mother or father or something. Not always, but a little bit."

Like Mitchell, she focused on her own sex in explaining why intercourse does not always lead to conception. He talked about the strength and number of sperm and the ages at which men produced them, while she centered, more accurately, on the availability of the egg: "They don't get a baby every time. It may be, like the middle of the month or something like that. Well, then the mother's not having her menstruation, and she can have a baby. But when she is, the egg can't be fertilized. Because it's just not in the right place or something like that. Or it's taken out. But when the egg is fertilized, it begins to grow and get bigger, to become a person, a baby, and then it gets big enough so that it comes out."

Both Mitchell and Tina show that even bright, knowledgeable, precocious early adolescents may not take into consideration all the factors leading to conception. In this way, they differ little from many adults. But what is most striking in their accounts of conception and birth is the absence of wonder. Naive and wanting to appear grown up, they keep any anxiety under control by talking about reproduction in terms of technicalities. The awe of the young child who sees birth as magical has gone underground, to surface again in the expectant parent. Few of the older children are ingenuous enough to admit that the facts they have worked so hard to understand are wonderful as well as true.

Physiology, love, marriage, religion, and the stork all figure in twelve-year-old Donna's account of sex and birth. More than any other child I spoke with, she was able to give each its due, recognizing the influence and weight of each factor without blending or confusing them. When I asked her how people get babies, she replied,

"Well, do you want the main thing? Well, they have sexual intercourse. And then the mother, when the egg is developed enough, she becomes pregnant by not having her period. And then she knows, and goes to a doctor, and they have all these tests. Then nine months the baby is developing, and by the seventh month, the baby can kick. It sucks its thumb and does things that it would usually do outside. And it can be born by seven months, but it is rather little. And by eight months the doctor usually says not to go anywhere out of Berkeley, out of wherever you live, not anyplace else. And by nine months you're supposed to stay really close to home. And you can't expect it on the exact date, but any time around that. Then the baby is born."

I asked her to define some of the words she used.

"*Born* means beginning a new life, or can mean beginning anything, I guess. The baby comes down a tube that opens down the vagina, and it's born!

"*Pregnant* means having somebody, something inside you, I guess. A baby.

"*Sexual intercourse*? Well, it should only be brought on by love, and it helps if you're married. And it's when the man and the woman come together, and the man sticks his penis into the lady's, near the womb, and then the egg that comes down through a little tube, down into the womb, is fertilized, and becomes a child."

Donna's description of fertilization uses an agricultural analogy to describe how children inherit their parents' traits. Her vivid images contrast with her hazy concept of what genes are all about: "Well, I guess it's just something that the man . . . Oh, wait, yeah, I know. All the things, like things that are going to be put into the baby, like what color hair it's going to be, if it's going to be curly and stuff, sort of like it gets fertilizer sprinkled on the little seed. It's sort of like the same idea, except instead of . . . bull . . . crap or whatever you might put on your plants, it's the genes, the way the baby's going to be after it's born. The genes are from the man and the woman. But when the man gives it to the woman, I guess it would be called the man fertilizing the woman." Clear that the egg "is not an embryo until it's fertilized," she had no preformist ideas.

Donna could take more than one perspective on the same events. Her theological explanation of the origin of babies did not contradict her description of the physiology of birth. Each point of view added to the full story of how people feel and behave to reproduce their own kind. When I asked her, "What is it about sexual intercourse that starts a baby?" she answered from several angles:

"Um, the fertilizing part, I guess. The part that a man and a woman love each other enough to have a child and to bring it into the world. If you want to think of the part that's the truth, or the mechanical stuff about it, if you want to think of the mechanical thing, the mother makes it. I don't know exactly, but if you were religious you'd say that God put it there. If you're religious you think that God put it there, because He wants another child on the earth, and that your love sort of sends a message, telling Him that you want a child. And if you're little, you tell a kid that the stork brings it. I always figured that the stork was God, and He's putting the child there. I guess that's how the word that the stork brings it got around. But a woman can't have a baby without having sexual intercourse, because the man has organs in him that have to go, or be put together with the woman's organs. If they're not put together, it's impossible."

Sex, love, God's will, early-childhood birth tales, and physiology are all there. The role of each is kept distinct and then fitted together so that none overshadows or engulfs another, showing that her conceptual skills are formal operational.

Her reminiscences about earlier thinking on the subject had an engaging, fanciful quality, incorporating images typical of the Level One Geographers and the Level Two Manufacturers: "Cartoons have lots of ways, but they're always, you know, that the stork brings them. Since I didn't have any little brothers and sisters when I was little enough not to understand, I didn't think about it. I just thought, you know, that it happened. A baby was there. Nothing ever started or anything. So I guess I just figured that you were there from the beginning of time, you know. Well, and once I saw a Shirley Temple movie, and everybody was up in the air, and all of a sudden a boat came by and the man would call out names. One time there was a couple of lovers there, and they had to be separated. You know, you were a big person, you grew up there. And when you grew up you started all over again. By the time you got down to earth, you were a child. It was just kind of. . . it was confusing to me. I didn't get it, but I guess that's how I figured it happened." The muddled and magical views of early childhood, while delightful, had left her, in her own words, confused. Some of the other older children had similar memories.

I asked all the eleven- and twelve-year-olds to try to remember how they used to think: "What did you think about how people get babies when you were little, before you understood it as well as you do now?" About two thirds of them could reconstruct the beliefs of earlier childhood, producing explanations that fit earlier levels in the sequence of stages I have been describing.

Ellen remembered believing that "babies just happened," and William "thought first that women just keep having babies and that birth control meant ways to keep them from getting them." James remembered thinking that babies were bought at the store. Although no child I spoke with, of any age, confessed to believing that storks delivered babies, three of the older children said that they used to think so when they were little. Kevin qualified this, stating, "I probably thought about the stork, that the stork brought them to the hospital probably." He thought he was four at the time. Tina remembered giving the doctor the critical role in conception, thinking that "the doctor had to do something to the mother at a certain time of the month."

Two children remembered thinking that a baby was a physical expression of the love between its parents. Susan believed that kissing produced babies, and Tessa, more abstractly, said, "I always thought that people were so much in love with each other that they just had babies, sort of like a reward or something for being in love with each other."

Karl recalled believing in the digestive fallacy, confusing conception with eating and birth with elimination "I think I thought that it grew up in her stomach from eating something special, and it came out when you shit in the toilet. I guess I was five or six then."

Jean, at twelve, described her beliefs about birth when she was six: "I thought that they went to a hospital, and the doctor put some medicine on the belly button, and the belly button would open up, and they'd take the baby out. And then they'd put the medicine back on, and it would close up, and then they'd have the baby."

Robert's memories were vivid. When I asked him if he remembered what he used to think, he answered in detail "Yes, I do. My sister said, 'I'm going to have a baby when I grow up.' And I said, 'You might not, it all happens by chance.' You know, all of a sudden, just BOOM, it comes out! I thought, see, my parents are lucky to have three kids. How come humans are so lucky that we have so many people in the world. I never learned, my mother and my father never told me about the birds and the bees, so, I went to school and I never got taught it. I just learned it from other kids. And then I got all my ideas changed. See, I had all these weird ideas about how you just got born by chance. You just quickly came out. Like when your mother goes to the bathroom, all of a sudden a baby falls out. And that's exactly what I thought. It's weird!"

These sixth- and seventh-graders find their earlier beliefs alien, "weird," and incomprehensible. Like adults, they have achieved some distance from their childhood ways of thinking and, having developed new problem-solving strategies and modes of thought, see the old ideas as so many cast-off, outgrown clothes, useless, amusing, or embarrassing—"Did I ever fit in that?"

Talking with Children

Knowing how children will eventually "put it all together" provides an approach to talking with youngsters who are almost—but not quite—there. In talking to Level Four Reporters and Level Five Theoreticians the objective is the same, although the Level Four child may take longer to understand why genetic material must unite to produce a baby. The Level Five child believes that the whole baby exists in either sperm or ovum, needing the other only to promote its growth. Children at these levels can be introduced to the idea that the baby has not begun to exist until the sperm and ovum meet and fuse. They can learn that the seeds of life come from both parents, from whom the baby inherits its physical characteristics.

A useful way to explain genetic contributions is to talk in terms of information. A parent might say that both sperm and ovum contain coded information about the baby they will grow to be. He can go on to talk about facial features, color of eyes, hair, and skin. It is important to stress that neither the sperm nor the ovum has the entire code until they unite. Together, they complete the message to develop into a baby that is the child of a particular set of parents.

For example, let's consider a conversation with a child who holds the Level Five theory that the baby is <u>really</u> in the sperm, needing the ovum only to feed and house the sperm as it develops into an embryo. A parent might encourage further speculation:

Parent: An interesting theory. Do you know what a theory is?

Child: Does it mean something that's not true?

Parent: No, a theory is an idea about how something happens that seems to fit the facts. It's an educated guess, by someone who's thought hard about the problem and has an idea that makes sense. A theory can be true, and a theory can be untrue. And sometimes we don't have enough evidence to decide.

Child: Is my theory true?

Parent: No, but it's a very good theory just the same. Not so long ago some of the very best scientists in the world thought about it just as you do. It wasn't until they had very powerful microscopes, so they could study how things happened very carefully, that they found out more about it. Can you think what they might have found?

Child: Was the baby really in the ovum?

Parent: What do you think?

Child: I don't think so.

Parent: You're right, it isn't. One way to think our way to how the baby is first formed is to think about how babies get to look the way they do, each one different. How do you suppose some babies get to have blue eyes and some babies are born with brown eyes?

Child: From their mother and father. I have red hair like

	Mommy, and everyone says my face looks just like yours, Daddy.
Parent:	I think so too. So if you grew from a sperm, it would be pretty hard to understand how you got all that red hair.
Child:	Something from Mommy must have got into me too. Something from the ovum, I guess.
Parent:	Uh-huh. Do you know what a code is?
Child:	Sure, that's special writing so only your friends know what you're saying. Little squiggles or numbers and things.
Parent:	Well, our bodies use a code to tell the baby how to develop. We call the little bits of coded information *genes*. There are genes that determine hair and skin and eye color, how tall we grow, whether our hair will be straight or curly, and lots of other things about how we look and how we'll grow. But each ovum and each sperm has only half the genes needed to start a baby. Until the sperm and the ovum join together, there isn't enough information about how to form a baby. When they're together, the code is complete and the message is to develop into a baby that is the child of this particular mother and father. Each baby is a new combination of their genes, so it looks a little like both but exactly like neither.
Child:	So the baby is <u>really</u> from both parents.
Parent:	Sure. We each get half of our genes from our mother and her ancestors and the other half from our father and his family. Neither the sperm nor the ovum can determine how the baby will grow on its own. But when they join together, they don't just get bigger, they form something entirely new: an embryo that will grow to be a baby.

Parents may want to include a discussion of how genes are arranged along tiny threadlike chromosomes in the nuclei of the sperm and ovum. Knowing that sperm and ova have only twenty-three chromosomes, while all other human cells have forty-six, gives children a mathematical handle on the concept that neither sperm nor ovum is complete and capable of generating new life on its own.

As they enter adolescence, children begin to think more about sexual matters, anticipating beginning to date and having to make decisions about how to behave sexually. With increasing rates of sexually transmitted diseases, including AIDS which is life-threatening, parents need to make sure that their youngsters understand the health consequences of sexual decision-making and how to reduce the risk of infection. Parents will probably want to be clear with their adolescent children about what their own standards of sexual morality are—and why they feel the way they do. Young people are more likely to embrace their parents' values when they understand that those values come from careful consideration of the issue and real concern for their children's growth and happiness, rather than fear and the arbitrary exercise of parental power. Only values which the adolescents have made their own, internalizing their parents' respect for them as self-respect, will have a lasting effect on their actions.

Information about conception and contraception do not encourage young people toward premature sexual activity. And ignorance is no deterrent. When more than 400,000 pregnancies occur each year among girls seventeen and younger, withholding information about contraception from teenagers is ridiculous. Because they can now differentiate between the physical, social, and moral aspects of sexual behavior, young people can (if they want to) understand that conception is possible even if the prospective parents (a) don't want a baby, (b) are not in love, and (c) are having sexual intercourse for the first time.

Talking about reproduction with young adolescents might well include thinking together about why people have children, as well as how they have babies. Parents will probably want to emphasize the importance of intention and planning in having children when one is ready to take care of them and help them grow. As with more factual matters, questions of value require that the discussion be a dialogue rather than a lecture. Young people are more likely to put into practice values that they participate in formulating. And lecturers are less likely to be consulted in time of doubt and confusion than people who state their positions clearly and who are truly responsive to the young person's feelings and thoughts.

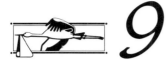

9

When the Doctor "Mostly Does Help"

A cartoon shows two children playing in a sandbox, comparing notes on their own origins: The first begins "My mother was a surrogate who had *in vitro* fertilization from an unknown donor sanctioned by my dad. How about you?" The other, in an aside, frets "I don't know if I can handle the laughter when I tell him the stork brought me!" (*Chicago Tribune*, April 9, 1987, p. 18)

Although it is seldom easy for parents to know what to tell children about sex and birth and when and how to tell them, the challenge is multiplied when developments in reproductive technology increase the complexities—physiological, technical, psychological, and ethical. "Surrogacy," writes political scientist Andrea Bonnicksen, "when combined with egg, sperm, and embryo transfer, creates streams of parental possibilities in which a child can end up with as many as five 'parents': a genetic mother, genetic father, gestational mother, social mother, and social father." But there is yet one more: since the law presumes that a woman's husband is her child's father, children born of married surrogates also have a "legal" father whose rights must be terminated to establish the parental rights of the man who may be both the social and genetic father. This addition of parents whose status requires explanation geometrically expands the complexity of the concepts involved. Even adults have trouble clearly understanding the myriad kinship possibilities, many of which are developmentally inaccessible to young children.

While language for building families via these routes is still evolving, two terms that describe procedures in a way that clarifies important distinctions have entered the lexicon. *Assisted reproductive technology*, or ART, refers to techniques for conception that require sophisticated medical technology. Examples are *in vitro* fertilization (IVF), gamete (ovum or sperm) intra fallopian transfer (GIFT), and zygote (or embryo) intra fallopian transfer (ZIFT). Artificial insemination using the husband's sperm (AIH), because it most often involves sperm washing and intrauterine insemination, is usually considered an ART. Donor insemination, however, can be done at home with a turkey baster with minimal training and without the help of any medical personnel, and is, therefore, not necessarily an ART. It is, however, a form of *collaborative reproduction*, a term coined by Elizabeth Noble to describe all those options that require the voluntary assistance of a person who will not parent the resulting child. Reproductive collaborators may donate ova or sperm, embryos that have been fertilized *in vitro*, or gestational capacity to a person or partnership who wish to initiate a pregnancy and parent a child. There can be assisted reproductive technology without collaboration, and collaborative reproduction without technological assistance.

Most often the use of extra-ordinary means for conceiving a child are prompted by medical circumstances. Infertile couples may choose to explore an array of possibilities, depending on the reasons for their infertility. The oldest form of collaborative reproduction, donor insemination, has been in use for about a hundred years and has led to the birth of approximately half a million children in the United States. (Lasker/Borg). Artificial insemination involves the transfer of a man's sperm to a woman's vagina, uterus, or fallopian tubes by nonsexual means. Typically, the ejaculate is introduced through medical intervention and fertilization takes place inside the mother's body.

The sperm used in artificial insemination may come from either the prospective father or a donor. Social acceptance for donor insemination, first successfully reported in 1884, has been slow in developing. As recently as 1954, an Illinois court ruled that artificial insemination by donor was adultery, the wife the adulteress, and the child a bastard of the illicit union. Since that time attitudes have changed remarkably, and now public acceptance of donor insemination for married couples has become fairly widespread. Traditionally, efforts are made to "match" the appearance, blood type, ethnicity, and sometimes even the interests and talents of the sperm donor with the prospective father.

In the past, when artificial insemination using only the husband's sperm (AIH) was unsuccessful, because of either a low sperm count or sperm with reduced motility, donor sperm was sometimes mixed with sperm from the prospective father to "boost" the chances of conception and add an element of ambiguity to the question of who is the genetic father. Mixing sperm is currently out of favor with infertility service providers, who believe that it represents a form of denial among those who have not yet come to terms psychologically with their infertility. In fact, it is considered poor practice by the American Fertility Society, which reports that inseminating with sperm from more than one man is also less likely to result in pregnancy.

In vitro fertilization (IVF), or fertilization "in glass", consists of bringing the reproductive cells together in a petri dish in the laboratory; the resulting embryo is then implanted in the uterus of the prospective mother. IVF may be limited to the parenting couple's own sperm and ova or involve a donor of male and/or female gametes. If a prospective mother has medical problems that preclude pregnancy, mother and father may arrange with another woman to carry the child to term. These "surrogates" are gestational mothers if they are implanted with embryos conceived *in vitro*, but they may also be genetic mothers if it is their own ova that are fertilized through artificial insemination with the prospective father's sperm.

The social realities of parents-to-be also necessitate medical or collaborative means of achieving conception. Increasingly, both single women without partners and lesbian couples have elected donor insemination as a way of forming a family. Less frequently, gay couples have arranged with "surrogate" mothers to bear the genetic child of one partner.

Earlier we saw that once children have been taught about how people get babies, it is sometimes difficult for them to understand why adults would have sex when they don't want a baby. It is still more difficult for them to comprehend the array of questions raised in a time when, to quote Brungs, we have "gone from sex without babies to babies without sex."

ART without Collaborators

We have come a long way from 1978 when newspapers around the world heralded the birth in England of "test tube baby" Louise Brown. *In vitro* fertilization no longer makes headlines, although newer ARTs and collaborative reproduction still generate controversy, as the ethical implications of each new development is explored, both seriously and sensationally, in the media. Between the time of each technological breakthrough and its popular acceptance, which is far from inevitable, there may be social stigma attached to means of reproduction that defy the notion of "doin' what comes naturally."

Discretion about such private matters is well-advised. People who are discomforted by ART, or merely curious, can be insensitive. Bonnicksen tells of a woman pregnant through IVF who told a co-worker she was going for a prenatal visit to her doctor and was asked, "What do they do? Check the tube?"

Until social thought and social policy catch up with varieties of family formation, care needs to be taken to protect against the dehumanization of children being labeled in terms of the medical procedures that their parents' utilized in having them. In *In Vitro Fertilization: Building Policy from Laboratories to Legislatures*, Bonnicksen urges that

"As citizens, we... heighten our feelings of control and responsibility by being vigilant about the imagery coming to us from different quarters. Test-tube babydom is an idiosyncratic image in an era of artificial organs and techniques. We do not talk about 'dialysis men' or 'valve women' or 'pacemaker persons' or use labels that marry people to techniques. We do not call premature infants 'incubated tots' or those born by caesarean section 'scalpel youngsters'... In the absence of data indicating children conceived externally are any different from other babies, one wonders if it serves any purpose to call them anything."

Six-year-old Denzel illustrates how the language Bonnicksen decries can lead to confusion in children. Denzel had already mentioned adoption and having sex as ways that people get babies, when I asked him if there are any other ways. "Inside a tube?" he responded tentatively. Asked what he meant, he explained that "You put the sperm in the tube." In describing pregnancy resulting from intercourse, he'd described how sperm and egg had to meet to start the baby growing. However, in describing growing a baby "in a lab," he omitted any mention of a female gamete, suggesting that after putting the sperm in the tube you just had to wait a long time "until it becomes a baby." Not yet fully operational in his thinking, he concretely pictures a "test-tube baby" who spends no time in a uterus and develops fully in the laboratory.

While they may create similarly literal ideas of *in vitro* fertilization, children this age and somewhat older can, with more information, be helped to understand that the embryo created by sperm and ovum in the laboratory must then be put into its mother's body to grow into a full-size baby and be born in the usual way. Understanding how and why this must be done, however, will remain difficult to grasp for years to come.

With a child created through *in vitro* fertilization using the parents' own sperm and ova, so that the parents she knows are her genetic parents as well, there may be no need to include the particulars of how she was conceived. As we saw in earlier chapters, children often assume that the baby is manufactured by putting together ingredients or components. The belief that medical intervention may be necessary to unite sperm and ovum is one that can occur spontaneously to children, who attribute extraordinary powers to doctors in their attempt to explain aspects of sex and birth that elude their grasp.

Remember Alice, for example, an In-Between who explained that "you need a mommy, a daddy, and a doctor to make a baby". According to this kindergartner, the doctor may furnish the seed and is indispensable, contributing "chemicals that help the baby grow," "situat(ing) the baby so it can grow and grow." Perhaps, she suggests, the doctor is also necessary to get "the stuff" out of the father and put it into the mother. Ursula, a few years older but also an In-Between, also mentioned medical assistance in conception, stating that there were pills "you take if you don't want a baby, and also there are pills you take if you do want a baby."

Most of the following discussion of children's need to know about their origins applies to not knowing a parent or having one or more social parents who are not their genetic parents. When there are two and only two parents involved, children do know all the significant personnel. Information about *in vitro* may be relevant at some point in their lives, but there is no deprivation involved in omitting the visits to infertility specialists. Just as parents deserve privacy in their sexual lives, which they do not and should not insist on imposing on their children, they need not feel impelled to disclose everything they have ever thought or done about infertility. Parents who have gone through onerous medical inventions may want their children to know how very much they were wanted and to tell them what parents had to go through to bring them into being. Care should be taken, however, not to burden the child, who may feel he has to be perfect in order to justify such extraordinary efforts. Parents need to ask themselves whether the information they are imparting is for the child's benefit or for their own.

Collaborative Reproduction: A Controversial Family Secret

Like adoption years ago, collaborative reproduction in forming families is shrouded in secrecy. As with adoption, too, children born

as a result of donor gametes or surrogacy have biological or gestational parents who do not raise them and whom they may not know.
As a result, openness about the way they were conceived is more
compelling than when genetic parents raise a child that medical
technology has assisted them in creating.

Efforts to study how children are affected by these new reproductive routes have met with insufficient response, as parents tend
to refuse researchers access to their children.[1] With heterosexual
couples, who until recently were the only people to whom these
options were made available and who have a choice about whether
to disclose the method of conception, doctors and therapists have
traditionally counseled secrecy. In donor insemination, the technique
with the longest track record, physicians kept the identity of sperm
donors secret, and advised couples not to inform friends and families about how they achieved pregnancy and not to tell their child
about her origins. Some doctors went so far as to recommend that
husbands not be told they were infertile or that donor semen had
been used in the procedure.

The reasons for secrecy were based on both legal and psychological grounds. Parents wanted protection from a donor who might
claim paternal rights or access, and donors wanted to be shielded
from unwanted obligations—financial or psychological—to the child.
Veiling the donor's identity was thought to offer some protection
against the "risk of fantasy," whereby the mother imagines a relationship with the man whose sperm has been used to inseminate
her, disrupting the marital bond. Protecting the father's self-esteem
was another vital consideration, with male infertility depicted as
more psychologically injurious than female responsibility for not
conceiving. Fathers of children born through donor insemination
sometimes talked about feeling "less of a man" or physically
defective, that they had let their wives down, and worried that the
children they went on to raise would be ashamed of their dads'
infertility. Fears about how a child would take the information were
probably the most compelling reason for secrecy: a child who doesn't
know there is an unknown genetic parent, it was reasoned, won't
feel driven to search for him and won't feel stigmatized as deviant
or abnormal. Why create unnecessary problems, this rationale

continued, as parents tried to put to rest any lingering shame or stigma in having required assistance in reproducing by avoiding conversations they expected would be awkward.

Until recently these arguments prevailed. Most studies of families using donor insemination reveal that the majority of parents do not plan to inform their children of the means by which they were conceived. A study by Judith Lasker and Susan Borg that queried infertility support group RESOLVE members, who might be expected to be more open about such matters than usual, revealed that slightly fewer than half planned to tell their children about donor insemination. A British study showed that only a few parents informed their children, and then only as adults. Too often children learned of their origins when their mothers, in the throes of marital battles, decided it was time they knew they weren't genetically related to their dads.

Fear of social censure or intrusive curiosity sometimes gives parents pause about how much to disclose about their child's origins. One mother, for example, decided not to discuss how she conceived her sons with anyone outside the immediate family upon learning that a friend had gone shopping with her newborn daughter only to overhear someone pointing to her and commenting "There's that artificial insemination baby."

Discretion in the community, however, is not the same as secrecy at home. Like adoption earlier, the tendency in families using collaborative reproduction is to be more and more open with children about their origins. Knowing one's genetic history, although still subject to debate, is more and more recognized as a right of the child, who cannot make informed medical decisions without this information. In their book *Lethal Secrets*, Annette Baran and Reuban Pannor cite evidence that a number of adult children conceived by donor insemination feel that their well-being has been adversely affected by not knowing. The most frequently mentioned source of distress is feeling that information central to their existence has been deliberately withheld from them.

Not every child will be affected in the same way by either knowing or not knowing. It is not the "facts" so much as what they mean to the individual that determines the emotional impact of this, or any, revelation. What is most destructive about keeping secrets is how it strains trust in relationships. This secret is especially central, bearing on the universal human question "Where do I come from?" If a child learns such important personal information from someone other than the parents, he may wonder if he has been deceived in other ways: might there be other secrets, lies, or misinformation between them?

It is not always possible to foresee how and when children will come across signs that they have not been been told an important part of the story. Visits to the doctor may raise questions about medical history that are met with discomforting silence, signaling something is amiss. Friends and relatives may unthinkingly comment with wonder on how a child conceived by donor insemination so closely resembles her father. Adults who discover this when they are grown have said that they suspected something all along and that finally being told brought them relief. While information can be troubling, suspicions can be more so.

The answer to the question—to tell or not to tell—is to inform the child, in ways that maximize understanding and minimize feeling deviant, but to be circumspect about who else you tell. One mother I called to interview in preparing this chapter was surprised that I knew about the circumstances of her son's conception. Had a mutual friend told me? No, I reminded her, she and her husband had told me thirteen years earlier, before the child's birth. She remembered getting more and more private as the years went by. During pregnancy and infancy, how he was conceived had been their story, but as he grew into childhood and adolescence the story was his, to tell or not to tell at his own discretion.

Although what a child is likely to understand at different ages should be an important part of judging how and when to inform children about out-of-the-ordinary means of conception and birth, parents' own emotional acceptance of how their family was formed is the first and most important step in preparing to talk with children. It takes careful attention and self-knowledge for reproductive pioneers to handle the emotional baggage of traveling beyond cultural frontiers. Insecurity can lead to destructive omissions, and inattentiveness to foisting unexplored and inappropriate expectations on the child. Because the child has been born through scientific intervention after long effort, she is welcomed with intense devotion and, perhaps, unrealistic demands. How can such a child be merely average!

In all instances when either or both parents are not the source of the child's genes, questions about the child's traits or behavior deriving from someone unknown pop up again and again. Parents' fantasies about an unknown gene donor can become a template for how they view their child. Because sperm donors, for example, are often medical students and residents, parents who are less educated or from a lower social class may have both higher ambitions for their child and mixed feelings about his achievements. On the other hand, parents may subscribe to a "bad seed" theory in explaining their child's less admirable traits, misconstruing normal misbehavior as evidence of an inborn defect.

Probably the most difficult emotional issue for parents, however, is when one of them is a genetic parent and the other isn't. Unlike the situation of adoptive parents, whose senses of legitimacy as parents are equal to one another, these families experience an imbalance in genetic parenthood that can have psychological consequences. When one parent feels more "legitimate" than the other, parent-child bonding can be affected; one parent may become significantly more attached to the child than the other, who may retreat both emotionally and from decision-making responsibility. In a worst case scenario, secrets about the other parent's not being genetically related have been used as ammunition in marital battles, sacrificing the child's welfare to a power struggle in the parental partnership.

Although it is best if these issues are carefully explored prior to making reproductive choices, there is no way to totally anticipate the ways they will reemerge, especially in conversations with children, whose questions can stir up old insecurities. It is vital for parents to check in with themselves periodically about how they are feeling about their reproductive choices, so that they can be thoughtfully attentive to the child's need when they are providing information and addressing concerns.

When Mommy AND Daddy Have a Collaborator

In families formed by male and female parents, children will not spontaneously raise questions about the role of collaborative reproduction in their conception and birth. While they may pick up on parental uneasiness in responding to the usual "where did I come from?" questions, they have no reason to assume extraordinary measures if there are no unexplained inconsistencies between the "facts of life" version of the origin of babies and the cast of characters in their own families.

In thinking about how to talk about collaborative reproduction, parents' decisions about what and how to inform their children will vary depending on family composition and the particular procedures involved. Nontraditional families will have no choice about early disclosure. For the very youngest children, different modalities of conception will figure prominently in talks between parents and children, because their thinking is very concrete and their focus is more likely to be on the mechanics of conception and birth. For older children, technical considerations recede. The questions which engage their hearts and minds have to do with what motivates people to participate in collaborative reproduction and how the special circumstances of their own coming into the world affect how they feel about themselves, their parents, and their search to figure out "Who am I anyway?"

Raising the Subject of Collaboration with Children

When Judith and Allan's son Jim was four years old, Judith was questioned by the mother of the boy's preschool playmate: "Do you have a friend who's a lesbian who has had a child? Your son told mine 'You don't need a man to have a baby, you just need a male friend to give you sperm.'" "Not my sperm," the second boy was reported to reply.

At the time of this anecdote, Jim did not know that he himself had been conceived through donor insemination. Because he had playmates who were the sons of lesbians, he had heard that the standard "facts of life" story had possible, nonstandard variations. A year later, in a conversation in which his mother explained how one of his friends had been conceived, she added "and we actually made you the same way."

More frequently, children born to heterosexual couples using donor insemination won't have friends from lesbian families to introduce them to this means of conception. For couples creating families under these circumstances, the topic of donor insemination can best be introduced as one of several means of uniting sperm and ovum. For example, in answering a child's question about how babies start to grow inside mothers' bodies, a parent might say:

Parent: Babies grow in the mother's uterus. To make a baby, grow, you need an ovum and a sperm. Women's bodies make ova, or egg cells, and men's bodies make sperm, which some people call seeds. To start the baby, a woman's ovum and a man's sperm must join together.

Child: How do they get together?

Parent: Sometimes the ovum and sperm get together when a woman and a man have sexual intercourse.* Sometimes a woman and a man try to start a baby, but a baby doesn't grow. There are lots of reasons why that can happen. Sometimes the reason is that the father's sperm can't join with the egg. Then, if they really want to grow a baby, they may get sperm from a man who gives his sperm so that people who want a baby very much can grow one in the mother's uterus.

Child: How does he give his sperm if they don't do intercourse?

Parent: When he has an orgasm,* the sperm come out of his penis into a cup. When he gives his sperm, he's called a sperm donor, or giver of sperm. He gives it to a place called a sperm bank that keeps it ready to use. Most of the time, doctors take the sperm and put it in the mother's vagina, so it can go meet the egg.

For many families, an obvious time to introduce information about donor insemination comes when they are attempting to conceive a subsequent child. When Paul was five, his parents took him along on trips to the fertility specialist. "What did the doctor do to you, Mommy?" he asked. His mother explained, "The doctor put the sperm in me. I had to stay on my back while the sperm swam to try to meet the egg." When he was seven, following his teacher's guidance that he was at an optimal age to receive more information about his own origins, his parents told him the "special story about how you came to us." His mother, an accomplished storyteller, wanted to spin a tale that would convey the love and magic that brought him into their lives.

His Daddy had had cancer as a young man, she reminded him, and it had been a very scary time. He'd been very sick, and the doctors had given him some very strong medicine that had killed the cancer cells, but the medicine had also killed some other cells. As a result, Daddy cannot make sperm," she told him. Sadly, he gasped, "Do you mean Daddy can't make any more sperm?"

His mother continued, telling him that they'd gone to a doctor who told them they couldn't grow a baby on their own, but that they could get some sperm from another man. Then after years of waiting and several tries, he began to grow. The story ended with his birth and his Dad's delighted exclamation "It's such a big boy."

"Can Daddy grow sperm again?" he asked. Told no, he looked serious for a minute, then said "Can you read to me now?"

"Does that mean Daddy's not my real father?" may be the child's next question. Telling a child, "I'm not your parent" is both untrue and destructive. Instead, a helpful answer could be "Daddy will always be your dad. It's just that Daddy's sperm didn't make you. The donor is your biological father." The issue of what makes someone a real parent is very similar to that in adoptive families, where it is also the case that the social parent is not the genetic parent. Reaffirming parenthood, followed by an exploration of the many ways to be a parent is the best response here, too. As with children who enter their families through adoption (see next chapter), children who were conceived through donor insemination might be asked "What do children's daddies do?", so that they can realize for themselves that daddies are clearly the fathers who take care of children.

For younger children, what is most needed is a reaffirmation of the parent-child bond. They want and need to know that a parent's commitment to them is unshakable, whether or not they are linked genetically. Later, when they are figuring out who they are and what it means to be like or unlike their parents in forging an identity that is their own, they will be interested in knowing more about who the genetic parent is and how their looks and personalities may derive from him or her. Adoption and infertility counselor Loni Hart suggests that heterosexual couples follow the example of single women and lesbians in asking sperm banks to disclose as much information about the donors as possible, so as to be able to answer their children's questions when they want to know more about that part of their genetic heritage.

Because preschoolers attribute so much power to people's wishes to be related, explaining that their mommies are their mommies "because I wanted her for a mommy" or "because she decided to be my mommy," they can conclude that their biological fathers have rejected them. "Why didn't the man who gave the sperm for me want to be my daddy?" they may ask. Here, the same kind of explanation that helps adopted children not feel personally rejected by their birthmothers can be brought to use. For example, a parent may respond to this question:

Parent: Your birthfather didn't know you, and he didn't know me. He gave his sperm to help make babies for people who really wanted babies but couldn't have them without his help. He didn't know who would get the sperm and even if a baby would grow when his sperm was used. He gave his sperm because he wanted to help out, not because he was ready to be a daddy to a child.

When Mother Is "Just Mommy"

Nearly a century after donor insemination became possible, ART developed to the point where women who could not conceive using their own ova might become pregnant using donated eggs for the first time. In 1988, ovum transfer resulted in successful conception and birth. When the prospective mother is pregnant with the child she will later raise, she is its gestational, as well as its social, mother. Because ovum transfer always entails *in vitro* fertilization, the child's daddy may or not be its genetic father, depending on the viability of his sperm.

If both donor ova and donor sperm are fertilized *in vitro*, the resulting pregnancy is called *embryo adoption*. Embryo adoption most often involves the implantation of an embryo which came from another couple's *in vitro* fertilization. When too many embryos develop to be safely implanted in the woman being treated, they may be available for other couples to "adopt." Although born to the mother whom he will know as mommy, the child whose origins include embryo adoption is nearly always genetically related to neither of his social parents, so that the dialogues for both donor insemination and ovum transfer will apply.

Discussing ovum transfer with children is analogous to explanations of donor insemination. The substitution of *woman* for *man* and *ovum* for *sperm* leads to almost identical conversations. The version of earlier explanations that applies in this circumstance is:

Parent: Sometimes the ovum and sperm get together when a woman and a man have sexual intercourse.* Sometimes a mother and father try to start a baby, but a baby doesn't grow. There are lots of reasons why that can happen. Sometimes the reason is that the mother's ovum can't join with the sperm. Then, if they really want to grow a baby, they may get an ovum from a woman who gives her ova so that people who want a baby very much can grow one in the mother's uterus.

After adopting her daughter, Amanda talked with her about her birthparents early in her life. Shortly after the adoption, she became pregnant with a son conceived using donor ova. When Mark was still a toddler, Amanda explained to him that "a part of my body didn't work right, and so another woman gave me what I needed for you to grow inside me." While the reference to "the woman who gave me what I needed" was somewhat more unwieldy than "birthmother," by the time he was three, he would point to anything oval in shape and declare "There's an ovum." Sometime in his fourth year, he told his mother "I understand it now. I grew inside another woman, and when I was ready to come out, they took me out of her and put me inside of you, so I could be born from you."

This way of understanding ovum donation is consistent with the Geographer's deeply held belief that he has always existed, and that the principal problem to be solved in fully accounting for his origins lies in where he happened to be before starting to grow in his mother's uterus. In Chapter Three, for example, Alexandra, explained that her little brother had been in a series of other women's tummies—because "only big girls can grow babies in their tummies—" before finally inhabiting the uterus of the mother who gave birth to him and brought him home to be a member of her family. Mark's mental picture, therefore, is not unique to his circumstances. He shares with his agemates an abiding belief that he has always existed, albeit in another location. The unusual part of his birth story is the involvement of a third party among the adults who created him.

Now six, he understands that the part of his mother's body called *ovaries* didn't work right and can't make ovum. He knows that doctors put his Daddy's sperm together with an ovum from another woman, and then put the combined sperm and ovum into his mother's uterus, where he grew for nine months until she gave birth to him. The part of the story that he is now most curious about is "How did they get the sperm out of Daddy to put inside you?"

Having learned about sexual intercourse, he knows that it is only one way that people go about having babies. Because young children frequently assume that their own experience is the norm, he frequently asks his mother "Did that person do sex to have the baby?" when they see a pregnant woman or a family with young children. One day he surprised Amanda by asking "In whose body did you grow?" "In Grandma's," she told him. "Did she do sex to have you?" he wanted to know. Told she had, he went on to probe further "Well, with who?" For Mark, Grandpa was one possible candidate, but not the obvious answer.

Discussions similar to those about what makes a parent a real parent both above and in the chapter on families who adopt their children can address children's questions about whether also having a genetic mother who has donated the ovum that led to their birth makes their mother any less real. The biological connection between mother and child during pregnancy and birth, however, goes a long way toward establishing her maternity. Contributing genetic material to the future child is only a small—albeit important—part of what mothers do to make babies, whereas for fathers it is their only biological contribution.

Perhaps the major difference in discussing the donation of ova, as compared with donor insemination, lies in how to refer to the child's genetic parent. *Birthfather* can be a useful term for a sperm donor—the role some birthfathers play in conceiving children is essentially to donate sperm, albeit directly. *Birthmother*, in contrast, is inextricably connected to the act of giving birth, so it would be misleading to use the term for a child conceived through ovum transfer or embryo adoption when his mother experienced both pregnancy and birth.

The solution to this problem may lie in the timing of the disclosure of donation. Children born through ovum transfer, unlike children born to single mothers or lesbian couples, do not present their parents with questions about their origins that necessitate talking about how they were conceived in the preschool years. For children with both a mommy and a daddy, perhaps the best time to introduce the special circumstances of their conception is in the early primary school years. The development of concrete operational thinking, typically at about seven years of age, allows children to begin to make sense of the terms *genetic mother* and *genetic father*, avoiding the confusion of introducing such complex concepts to still younger children. Delaying confiding this information still later, however, runs the risk of adding to the emotional turmoil set in motion by puberty. While children may not be able to cognitively assimilate all the complexities of collaborative reproduction, even in middle childhood, those who are not told until they are adolescents or adults are more likely to be angry at having been kept in the dark about their origins.

Surrogacy

Surrogacy, whereby a woman intentionally agrees to become pregnant with a child she plans to give to someone else to parent, is so recent a development that less is known about how children will think and feel about joining their families in this way. (While ovum transfer and embryo adoption are also very new, the analogy to donor insemination sheds some light on how children are likely to feel about them.) Like many children who were adopted at birth, most children born to surrogate mothers will have grown inside the body of someone whom they probably do not know. Unlike adopted children, however, they have been born from a woman who planned to serve as a carrier only, making an adoption plan before intentionally conceiving, and, in most instances, they will grow up with their biological fathers. The principal difference for the child is in understanding the adults' motivations in arriving at a surrogacy plan.

Reasons for using surrogate mothers to create families vary. For some women, pregnancy may entail extraordinary risks to life or health. Before the development of ovum and embryo transfer, surrogacy was the only alternative to adoption when the reason for a woman's infertility was the nonviability of her ova. Nor can all female infertility be remedied by the use of donor ova. When a woman has an illness that makes pregnancy hazardous or has had a hysterectomy, for example, having another woman carry the baby to term is the only means of having a child genetically related to at least one parent.

There are two types of surrogacy. In *gestational surrogacy*, a couple's own gametes are fertilized *in vitro*. The resulting embryo is then introduced into the uterus of the surrogate mother, who carries the baby to term and gives birth. Because the parents who will raise the child are his only genetic parents, a court order can be obtained that permits them to be listed on the birth certificate, and there is no need for legal adoption. While she is neither the source of the child's biological heritage nor the mommy who takes care of him day to day, a woman who has a baby grow inside her body for nine months and then gives birth is a mother, too. Hillary Hanafin, of the Center for Surrogate Parenting in Beverly Hills, suggests *birthing mother* may be the best way to refer to gestational surrogates, especially with young children, while Susan Cooper and Ellen Glazer argue, in *Beyond Infertility*, for the term *gestational carrier*.

In *artificial insemination surrogacy*, the surrogate mother is inseminated with the sperm of the prospective father, so that it is her ovum that is fertilized. She is, therefore, both the genetic and the gestational mother to the child, who must then be legally adopted by his intended mother. Describing the surrogate mother's relationship to the child is very much like with adoption, differing only in that the adoption plan was made prior to conception rather than as the result of an ill-timed pregnancy. Much of the information in that chapter will be useful. In talking with the child about how he came into being, the term *birthmother* is an appropriate one. For all children born through surrogacy, however, using first names to identify the women who gave them birth will probably be the most frequent, accessible terms of reference.

A child born to a surrogate mother may be the genetic child of neither, one, or both of the parents with whom he makes his home. Regardless of his genetic heritage, the topic will usually emerge when he learns that babies grow inside mothers' bodies and talks with his mommy about when he was in her tummy. This is a time to gently introduce the subject of his particular way of entering the family:

Mother: It would have been wonderful if you had grown in my uterus, but I can't grow babies in my uterus. We wanted to have a baby very, very much, so Daddy and I looked and looked until we found a very special woman who agreed to help us grow a baby.

The next part of the story will depend on whose ovum and whose sperm were involved. When, as is probably most frequently the case, the father's sperm were used to inseminate the surrogate mother, the parent might continue:

Mother: So the doctor put Daddy's sperm in the woman's vagina. His sperm joined with one of her eggs, and she became pregnant with you. You grew inside her uterus until you were big enough to be born. We were so happy when you were born. We thanked (birthmother's name or "your birthmother") over and over for helping us have you. Then we took you home and named you (child's name) and loved you very, very much.

When both parents are the source of the child's genes, the story is somewhat different:

Mother: You grew from Daddy's sperm and my ovum, but my

uterus wasn't a place where a baby could grow. So the doctor helped put the sperm and the ovum together, and then she put you inside (surrogate's name or 'your birthing mother's') uterus. She took very good care of you during the nine months you grew inside her body. Then when you were ready to be born... (as above).

Children as young as three or four can understand that they have extra-ordinary origins "because Mommy's body didn't work for growing babies." Saying "Mommy's tummy was broken" may seem more accessible to young children, but it is less specific and more suggestive of damage that may trouble some children. Like children who are adopted, children born through surrogacy may mourn not being born from the mother they know and love. Three-year-old Anita, for example, asked, "Mommy, please can I climb up you and crawl back out. Then I can say I came out of you?"

Learning about having had a birthmother or birthing mother may invite more questions. Six months after being told about her "special beginnings," four year old Jenny said, "Mommy, I want to know more about Carole." Her mother took down an album of photographs of the birthmother's family, which included pictures of her daughter's halfsiblings. Jenny seemed most interested in the dog, and, her curiosity assuaged, she moved on to other activities. When young children are assured that their questions can be answered without creating parental consternation, they seem to accept information with relative equanimity.

When a younger sibling is also born through surrogacy, children can be matter-of-fact about situations that give most adults pause. During the pregnancy that led to her brother's birth, four year old Anita went with her mother and the baby's birthmother for prenatal checkups. "I came out of Mindy's tummy," she told friends and acquaintances, "because my Mommy's tummy doesn't work right. My baby brother is going to come out of Susan's tummy at Easter time."

Parents of children born through surrogacy struggle with how much to use the word *adoption* in talking with their children. In the case of gestational surrogacy, this term is misleading, because the child is living with both genetic parents. When this is not the case, however, some information about the legal adoption is a necessary assurance to the child that her relationship with her mother is an irreversible one. A mother might then follow the story of the child's birth with "and then I adopted you, so that everyone would know that I was your Mommy forever and ever."

"Well, I'm sort of adopted," said Elena, a six-year-old whose maternal aunt is her genetic mother. "My aunt's my mom," she started to explain, only to later correct herself, sorting out the complexity of the resulting relationships: "Well, my Mom's my mom, and my cousins are sort of my sisters." Even when family members are surrogate mothers for a relative's child, children are very clear that the people with whom they live, the mommy and daddy who take care of them, are their "real," psychological, parents.

Tina, at eight, was told by her parents that her Aunt Jean, who was also her birthmother, would "take care of you if anything happens to us." Tina, who knew that Aunt Jean had given birth to her, protested "But I don't even know her." Reticent about talking about her origins, even with her parents, she later surprised them by responding to an assignment on the theme "I am special because..." by writing "I am special because my real mother couldn't have a baby, so my aunt had me for her."

Another question that vexes many parents, according to Hanafin, is how to talk with children about their biological halfsiblings. Nearly all surrogate mothers already have children, but few parents of children born through surrogacy volunteer to their children that they have halfsisters and -brothers who live with the birthmother.[2] This reticence usually stems from concern that the child will then feel somehow less theirs, as if knowing that there are other children to whom the child is also related will make him feel less connected to the family he lives with. For preschoolers, whose concept of family is based primarily on sharing a household, this is not an issue—one way or the other.

When Anita's little brother was born, she went to the hospital to greet him. His birthmother's four children were also there. "We're the Three Musketeers," announced four-year-old Anita and six-year-old Steven, as three-year-old Michael nodded in agreement, "and we're going down the hall to see our baby brother." Later,

Anita told Steven, "He's not your brother." Anita's mother corrected her: "He's also Steven's brother." But Anita is convinced that the baby is more her brother than theirs: he lives in her house, and his mommy is her mommy.

As they become older and cognitively more mature, biological and legal considerations will weigh more heavily in their thinking about who is family to them. While parents may want to downplay genetic sisterhood or brotherhood, it is essential to respond to questions honestly and give children permission to count their half-siblings in or out of the family roll call, depending on the child's needs—be they developmental, existential, or idiosyncratic. The chapter on stepfamilies may provide a useful approach.

Why Become Pregnant with a Child When You Won't Be Her Mommy

Because it will seem obvious to them why their parents very much wanted them to come into the world, why parents seek recourse in collaborative reproduction is easier for children to understand than why the other parties to the arrangement agree to participate. In middle childhood their curiosity about the motivations of ovum and sperm donors will become more of an issue, but for preschoolers the psychosocial implications of donating genetic materials are too abstract to capture their attention for long. For now they seem satisfied with altruism or generosity as sufficient motive. The question of why a woman would agree to be impregnated and carry to term a baby she had no intention of parenting may be more difficult for them to pass over in the early years. The time it takes, the physical closeness of birthmother and fetus, and the ordeal of labor and birth, raise the same questions that occur to adopted children who wonder why a birthmother would make an adoption plan.

The questions may be the same, but the answers are very different. In the next chapter, we will see that adopted children in the preschool and early elementary years focus mostly on how youth and poverty lead some women with unplanned pregnancies to make an adoption plan before the birth of the babies they will later deliver. Faced with very limited and difficult choices, the birthmother whose baby is later adopted selects among the few alternatives to do the best she can, both for the baby and for herself. With surrogate mothers, however, becoming pregnant on behalf of others is a choice made more electively under less accidental circumstances. In responding to children's "whys", one possible explanation is:

Child: Why did my birthmother have a baby if she didn't want to be my mommy?

Parent: Most birthmothers who help mothers and fathers have babies already have children. They know how wonderful it is to have a child to love and take care of, and they want to help people who can't have a baby start a family. Sometimes they have a sister or a close friend who's tried to have a baby and wasn't able to, so they knew how important it was to us to have you. Also, women who decide to be birthmothers usually really like the feeling of being pregnant and would like another chance to be pregnant, even if they already have as many children as they want to parent.

"Why did she have me?" five and a half year old Jenny asked her mother, as she wondered for the first time about the motives of her birthmother. Her mother answered along the lines suggested above: "Carole, your birthmother, had two children. She didn't want any more children to parent, but she wanted to help people who couldn't have a baby on their own." She made clear to Jenny that Carole had participated in planning for her birth. "You know, Mommy," Jenny volunteered, "I really love Carole." When asked why, she continued "Because she let me be born."

Explanations that satisfy younger children will not always continue to be sufficient as time goes by. Especially when the surrogate mother is also the genetic mother, older children will return to the question of how she came to her unusual decision. As they become more savvy to the ways of the world, they may suspect that there are aspects of the arrangement that altruism does not explain. Because money changes hands in most surrogacy contracts, a child may struggle with how to think about the financial exchange without seeing either himself or the birthmother as a commodity. While surrogate mothers are not always economically less well off than the

couples with whom they contract, the challenge is to present the
economics of surrogacy without creating a picture of the surrogate
mother as either mercenary or exploited.

Child: You mean you hired her to get pregnant and give birth?
She did it for the money?

Parent: Being pregnant and giving birth takes a lot of energy and
a lot of time, and it involves discomfort. Especially in late
pregnancy, it is hard to work at other jobs. It's only fair
that someone be paid for her time and effort. But while
your birthmother needed to be taken care of during her
pregnancy, money wasn't the main reason she did it.
There are lots of easier ways to earn money. And the
doctors (or agency) who helped us take a lot of time to
make sure that the women they find really want to help
people who can't have babies on their own and are not
just in it for the money.

"It's Not Our Baby, It's Jack and Karen's Baby"

Because having already had children is frequently a criterion
by which surrogate mothers are selected, children whose mother
elects to be pregnant with a child who will live in another family
must also make sense of this innovative reproductive turn of events.

"Are you pregnant with twin Japanese babies?" Janet was
asked by her son's kindergarten teacher, who was sure that five year
old Kevin's contribution to Show and Tell was so farfetched that it
might just be true. Similarly, eight-year-old Beth startled the congre-
gation by asking their minister "Would you please say a prayer for
my little sister in Chicago?", prompting her parents to worry that
their spiritual leader would wonder which one of them might be
unfaithful.

The mothers of both of these children were surrogates collabo-
rating in building other families: Janet was a gestational carrier for a
Japanese couple, while Beth's mother, Ellie, was the birthmother for
a family who lived hundreds of miles from their home. Ellie had told
Beth and her brother, Jimmy "We've met a couple named Jack and
Karen. Jack and Karen cannot have a baby from Karen's belly, so
Mommy is going to help them have a baby. I only wanted two chil-

dren. Beth and Jimmy, you are the only two children I want to raise. So, I am going to help Jack and Karen bring a baby into the world, and then the baby will go home and be their baby."

Five at the time, Beth surprised her mother by stating matter-of-factly, "Well, if you couldn't have children, you'd have someone else have them for you." Later, when people would ask, "When is your baby due?" Beth would reply, "It's not our baby—it's Jack and Karen's baby." Because Ellie and her husband felt that they had made a good decision about her being a surrogate mother, they felt that their children accepted it as normal. "I think it's taught them an indirect lesson—that it feels good for us as a family to help another family."

Prospective surrogates with older children are counselled to include their children in the decision-making. They are encouraged to first explain surrogacy, then ask for the children's feelings about what it might mean for them: "Mommy wants to do this, but it's a family decision." Christie Montgomery, of Surrogate Parenting Services and a former surrogate herself, reports that children's attitudes reflect those of the adults in their lives. It is, therefore, essential to their own children's best interests that prospective surrogates resolve any lingering conflicts before becoming pregnant. Montgomery cautions, "It is traumatic to tell children 'This is your sister, and we have to give her away'."

Collaborative Reproduction in Nontraditional Families

Children begin by assuming that their own experience is universal. When they don't have either a father or a mother, these words may not conjure up a mental picture. They hear other children use a word, but they may not be clear about what it means. Susan, a lesbian mother, remembers that her oldest son, at eighteen months, attended a daycare in which the children would congregate at closing time, putting on their coats and waiting for parents, mostly fathers, to pick them up. For a short time, she recalls, he thought a daddy was a coat. Similarly, a married father whose toddler called him *Papa* found that his son's nursery school playmates, who were from homes in which fathers were called *Daddy*, thought Papa was his first name. When he arrived to pick up his son, he would be met with a chorus of "Hi, Papa."

Understanding that a word used as a name can also describe a category of people can be especially confusing to preschoolers. At three, the daughter of a gay couple called one of her two fathers *Daddy* and the other *Papa*. When told "You have two daddies," she'd protest "No, I have one Daddy and one Papa." A year later, she understood that daddy could describe a relationship as well as being the way she addressed one of her parents.

For the children of always-single parents and same-sex couples, questions about the "missing" parent arise when they begin to recognize that people come in two sexes and that most families include both male and female adults. This usually occurs late in the third or early in the fourth year of life, when questions are likely to be a variant of "Do I have a daddy?" Susan reports that her son Bill seemed to feel that because he had two parents, although both were mommies, he was like everyone else. Then, at age three, he asked, "Do I have a daddy?" It wasn't until he was almost four, and she was pregnant with her second child, that he wanted to know how his two mommies had been able to have a child without a daddy. At that time, Susan reports, "I told him that I wanted to have a baby and there was a very nice man who gave us the sperm and we put them inside."

Telling children that they have two mommies or just a mommy, two daddies or just a daddy, is an important part of their family story. It's important, also, to add that they have a birthmother or a biological father, so that they know how to respond when other children tell them in no uncertain terms that it is impossible to have a baby if you don't have both a mother and a father. Of course, the absence of a mother will need more explanation than the absence of a father among young children who have not yet connected the father with pregnancy and birth. Schoolyard—even nursery school—discussions of this topic occur much sooner than most parents expect, so some mention of the other biological parent needs to be part of the story of a child's origins early on.

For most single mothers by choice and lesbian couples, donor insemination is the route to family formation. Children born to single mothers and lesbian couples will want and need to know about donor insemination before similarly conceived children of heterosexual couples. As we learned above, the first question a child is likely to ask is "Do I have a daddy?"

One way to respond to the question is to distinguish between daddies and fathers, perhaps borrowing the term *birthfather* from the adoption literature. Although *genetic father* is more accurate, the concept is a difficult one, and probably can best be introduced during the primary school years.

Parent: You have a mommy (or two mommies). You don't have
            a daddy, but you do have a birthfather. Your birthfather
            is the man who gave his sperm so that I (we) could have
            you, because all babies start when a sperm from a man
            joins with an ovum from a woman.

It is helpful if a mother can go on to answer questions, to the extent of her knowledge, about her child's father. Because children's thinking is closely tied to what they perceive in concrete images, the more descriptive details available, the more able they are to construct a satisfying internal image. Even when, as is most often the case, the sperm donor is anonymous, biographical information is often available to fill in the child's mental picture.

"How come I don't have a daddy?" can be answered in terms accessible to preschoolers, who frequently see people as related to each other because they want to be. Single mothers might answer: "I wanted very much to be a mommy, but I didn't know anybody I loved enough to live with and make a family with." Lesbian couples, on the other hand, can explain that their love for each other led them to want to create a family together, so their child has two mommies, instead of a daddy and a mommy.

Not all donors, however, are anonymous. Single mothers and lesbian couples are more likely than heterosexual couples to locate donors on their own. Parents and donor can then contract among themselves as to the degree of contact between father and child or whether the father wants to be known to the child or not. At one end of the continuum, a lesbian couple and a gay couple may agree to coparent, in joint physical and legal custody, the offspring of one woman and one man. The range extends to include fathers who have intermittent contact with their children, who are raised primarily by their single mothers or lesbian parents, or those who simply supply information so that their offspring can contact them when they become adults and elect to meet a heretofore unknown genetic parent. The tendency is for there to be increasing information and accessibility, in response to adult children's reports of psychological distress in being denied access to their genetic histories.

In talking with children about the origin of babies, parents can introduce the use of donor sperm along with sexual intercourse as alternate means of arranging for the union of sperm and ovum. For example, in answering a child's question about how babies start to grow inside mothers' bodies, a parent might say:

Parent: Babies grow in the mother's uterus. To make a baby grow, you need an ovum and a sperm. Women's bodies make ova, or egg cells, and men's bodies make sperm, which some people call seeds. To start the baby, an ovum from a woman and a sperm from a man must join together.

Child: How do they get together?

Parent: Sometimes the ovum and sperm get together when a woman and a man have sexual intercourse*. OR (Single mother version) When a woman really wants to be a mommy and she hasn't found someone she wants to be her baby's daddy, she may get the sperm from a man who gives his sperm to help women have babies. OR (Lesbian couple version) When two women love each other and want to start a family together, they may get the sperm from a man who gives his sperm to help women have babies.

Child: How does he give his sperm if they don't do intercourse?

Parent: When he has an orgasm*, the sperm come out of his penis into a cup. When he gives his sperm, he's called a sperm donor, or giver of sperm. He gives it to a place called a sperm bank that keeps it ready to use. Most of the time, doctors take the sperm and put it in the mother's vagina,

so it can go meet the egg. Sometimes, the mother
(or mothers) put it in the vagina herself.

Children told by their mothers about the process of donor
insemination have a rudimentary grasp of the essentials. Thomas,
eight, and Katrina, seven, are each the only child of single mothers,
who have talked with them about their being conceived through
donor insemination.

"How do people get babies?" I asked Thomas. "The sperm
bank," he quickly responded, "or a husband." I asked him to tell me
more about each: "Well, with the sperm bank, you go to the sperm
bank and ask for a jar of sperms. That's how my mommy got me."
According to Thomas, the mother pours the sperm into her vulva,
after which she will usually have a baby in a couple of years. He
understands that sperm and ovum need to come together to start a
baby and that the alternate route to conception, mentioned second,
is for the husband to "squirt the sperms out of his penis into his
wife's vulva. That's the other way."

Less forthcoming than Thomas, Katrina was reluctant to
answer how the sperm and egg get together to create a baby. After a
long pause, I asked her if there was more than one way. "There's
two," she replied, going on to describe her own conception but pre-
ferring not to describe sexual intercourse: "Well, the way my mom
got me... I have a father, but I don't know him. She wasn't married
to him. She went to some kind of place that had sperms, but no
man. She took home the sperms and... I'm half Latino and my
father's Latino. And she took one of the sperms and she had me."

Katrina was quick to point out that her mom "didn't have sex."
Asked how her Mom had decided to have her that way, she replied
"She never wanted to marry a man, to have a baby by sex."

Children's early understanding of the motivation for collaborative reproduction involves answering for themselves both why a parent chooses to have a child in this way and why a donor chooses to
collaborate in building another's family. Most children will assume,
even if they have not been told, that their parent chose to bring them
into the world by whatever means they have done so. Like Katrina's
mother, who told her "I wanted to have a child, but I didn't want to
be married," parents can help their children feel good about their

origins by letting them know that they have built a family in the best way available to them. The motivation of the unknown donor is more elusive. Because his identity is often masked, children can only speculate as to what led him to his decision. Asked why men give their sperm to sperm banks, Katrina answered "sometimes they don't want to be fathers, but they want to help women who want to be single mothers." Thomas' explanation of how the sperm bank gets sperm was somewhat less altruistic: "They buy it...from the employee." Puzzling over why donors may offer their sperm, he was visibly relieved when I made a suggestion, something I rarely do, that they want to help people who can't otherwise have families. "I think so, too," he grinned. His relief bespeaks the need children have for the story of their origins to be benevolent and loving.

For gay couples, the more obvious need for a surrogate mother means that children will be informed even earlier about this way of forming families. As in homes without a father, the child's first question is likely to be about the missing parent: "Do I have a mommy?" A father might respond:

Father: You have two daddies. You don't have a mommy, but you do have a birthmother, because all babies grow inside mothers' bodies. We wanted to have a family very much, so we found a woman who agreed to be pregnant with you. I gave some sperm that the doctor put in your birthmother's vagina, and you began to grow, just as every baby starts when a sperm from a man joins with an ovum from a woman. Then after nine months, you came out your birthmother's vagina, and we thanked her very much and named you...

Gay couples report that casual encounters with bystanders often lead to comments about their child's mother. A man out with a very small child is often greeted with "Oh, Mom's day off" or "Aren't you nice to be helping your wife?" In contrast to children who live with their mothers, children of gay men are continually confronted with questions prompted by strangers' mistaken assumptions about their families. Even before the child might be spontaneously curious, she will be called upon to field questions about her mommy. At three, Delia, the daughter of one gay couple, became adept at responding to such remarks with "I have a birthmother." Her friends, too, understand that "Delia has a birthmother." Her daddy thinks her preschool playmates may think of her as having been adopted.

Told about her birthmother before she was three as the special "someone who helped us create you," it has become an important component of Delia's understanding of the ways in which her family is both the same as and different than other families. The family has occasional contact with her birthmother, who is clearly a figure of some interest to her, entering into her fantasy play. Overhearing her talking about "My old mom and my old dad," her fathers were amused to learn that she imagined the latter to be President Clinton.

Delia also demonstrates how children's experience in their own families can often be disregarded as they are inducted into the social expectations of their culture. Like children who insist that "dads go to work and moms take care of children" even when their own parents have not followed these conventional sex role prescriptions, Delia disregards her own experience when it contradicts social convention. "Two women can't get married," she protested when told the family would be attending a lesbian wedding. When they arrived at the site for the ceremony, Delia repeatedly asked "Where is the ship?" Having derived her concept of marriage from *The Little Mermaid*, she thought that all weddings occurred on shipboard.

It is important that parents of children who were conceived collaboratively, especially those whose family constellation obviously leaves something to be explained, find out what the schools are teaching and coordinate the introduction of information. A lesbian mother who made a point of talking with the teacher who would be addressing her son's class testified as to how helpful it was for the teacher to include donor insemination in her presentation to the children. "It's essential," she emphasized, "to make the environment as inclusive and normative as possible. I let the teacher know so that education could come from the educators. It's important that adults educate the kids, so that our children aren't responsible for doing all the educating."

Talking with Children as They Grow

So far, I've addressed how to talk with young children about the mechanics of conception and birth when there are genetic or gestational parents they do not know. As with other aspects of children's sex education, these will not be one time conversations. The concepts are complex and will take time to assimilate. Along the way children may mix things up. One nine-year-old girl born to a lesbian couple through donor insemination told her therapist "My father is a scientist," confusing the scientific procedure which led to her conception with the occupation of the sperm donor.

Sometimes parents think information has been absorbed, only to discover that a child's understanding was, at best, partial. Sheila's mother was surprised to hear her eleven-year-old ask "Do you and Dad use condoms?" because Sheila had been told years before that she had been conceived through donor insemination. "Don't you remember Daddy doesn't have any sperm?" mother replied. "Then how can he be my daddy?" Sheila demanded.

It is helpful to check in with them from time to time, asking perhaps "Do you ever think about your birthfather?" or "Do you have any questions about how you were born?" The challenge here, as it is with adoption, is to strike a balance—letting them know you're open to their concerns without insisting that they must feel different.

Their questions about the nuts and bolts of how things work having been answered, children's interest in these issues tends to follow the same course as when adopted children are assimilating the story of their own origins: why do some people require special assistance in creating families, why do other people donate their sperm or ova, and what would make a woman want to carry a child to term when she knows before she even gets pregnant that she will not mother that child? Still more pressing is how their atypical beginnings affect who they know themselves to be: "What does it mean about *me* that I have genetic parents elsewhere whom I may not know?"

Why Collaboration Was Necessary

Children's questions about why their parents had to take atypical measures to conceive may be difficult to answer. Infertility, even when it is treated successfully in the end, leaves its wounds. Children's probes can touch on delicate topics that evoke unresolved pain, anger, and insecurity. Parents would do well to take the time to explore for themselves what they want to say to their children about the need for assistance in reproducing before questions arise. One mother of a child born through surrogacy started practicing telling her daughter about her origins when she took her home from the hospital. By the time the little girl was old enough to understand, she reasoned, her mommy would be comfortable telling the story.

Careful thought is needed to say neither too little nor too much. Saying too little leaves big gaps in the puzzle, leading both to confusion and a sense that something is being avoided. Saying too much, going into detail about the frustrations of years of infertility treatment, on the other hand, places an undue emotional burden on the child.

When there are clearcut medical reasons for needing reproductive collaboration, a child can be given a brief version of the facts tailored to her level of understanding. For example, in explaining the need for donor sperm, a father might say:

Father: Some sicknesses hurt the sperm so they can't be used for making babies. When I was already grown up I got sick with mumps, which made it so we needed to get some sperm from another man.

If early menopause is the reason why ovum transfer was done, a mother might say:

Mother: My body stopped making egg cells. Every woman is different, but most go on to make ova for a few more years. When I found out that I couldn't make ova anymore, Daddy and I decided to see if we could get ova from a woman who would help us by giving us some of hers.

Because sperm and ova are less visible than the enlarged abdomen of a pregnant woman, younger children are more likely to question why the mother could not be pregnant. Again, if the answer is simple and straightforward, they can be given the short version of the medical story. As one example, "You know I once had a sickness called cancer. A lot of doctors think it is dangerous for women who had that sickness to be pregnant. I'm not sick anymore, but I was told not to get pregnant because I might get very, very sick. But women who didn't have that disease don't usually have that problem." But if it pertains children can also be told "We don't know exactly why, it just didn't work for a baby to grow there."

In thinking about what led their parents to need unusual assistance in reproducing, one vital concern for children is whether they, too, will be able to have babies only with special technical aid. Identifying closely with their parents, children are likely to assume that they will follow in their parents' footsteps in this, as in many other ways. They need to learn that almost all causes of infertility are not hereditary, so that the chances of being infertile are not very different for them than for anyone else.

How Can They Give Away Part of Themselves?

As children begin to think more abstractly as they approach puberty, their attention may return in a more probing way to the sperm or ovum and their unknown donors. More aware of what it is about the sperm and ovum coming together that creates new life, they may find it harder to understand how someone can donate such a vital part of themselves and seem disinterested in the child that may result from such a gift.

Knowing, for example, that a donor probably has no idea of how many children were helped into being by his visits to the sperm bank, or who or where they are, may not answer their concern when what they are struggling to come to terms with is a casualness toward genetic progeny. In a study by Joseph Davis and Dirck Brown, one child born of donor insemination complained: "I wanted to know how he could have sold what was the essence of my life for $25.00 to a total stranger, then walk away without a second thought... Why couldn't he connect the semen to the human being it would create?" (p. 156, in Lasker and Borg)

Preteens and teens raise some of the same questions as medical ethicists who argue for the decommercialization of reproductive technology. Whether the sum is minimal, as for sperm, or considerable, as for gestational motherhood, it is discomforting to think of oneself as a commodity. Their other primary concern is the presumed disinterest of the gamete donor. It may be somewhat reassuring to learn that just as children have fantasies about their genetic parents, so, too, do donors have fantasies about their offspring, whom they continue to think and wonder about.

A parent could address the concerns expressed by the girl quoted above:

Parent: It would be nice if we could know everything he thought and felt about being a sperm donor. I'd like to think he takes pleasure in having made it possible for you to be born and for us to be a family, that sometimes when he goes to sleep at night he wonders who might have been born from his sperm and what you might be like. I don't know that he does, but I also don't know that he doesn't. I do know that many men who donate sperm do think about the children that they may have helped bring into the world.

Egg donors are usually selected more carefully, in part because of the invasiveness of the procedure necessary and in part because of the greater investment women are seen as having in their reproductive lives. It is harder to think of an ovum donor as casual about her contribution. This very lack of casualness, however, may make it hard for a child to understand how a genetic mother could have no connection to him. It might be helpful to talk about how grownups, too, can find the connection between a reproductive cell—sperm or ovum—and an actual, living, breathing child to be more than a little abstract. A parent might say:

Parent: I know it's hard to understand how someone who had so much to do with making you who you are—giving you half your genes—could help create you and then not want to go on being part of your life. I think sometimes people have a hard time holding all those possibilities in their minds. It's hard, sometimes, for a man to imagine that one of the billions of sperm his body makes actually ends up as half of what becomes a real, live baby, or for a woman to think that one of the egg cells taken out of her body actually becomes part of a baby that grows inside another mother. You know, both men and women who donate sperm or ova often don't know if their cells lead to a successful pregnancy. They may like the idea of helping others start families and not have a really clear idea in their minds of how to think of a child who may or may not exist. I know some donors think 'Well, I wasn't planning on using this ovum/sperm anyway, so if I can help someone else in this important way, I'd like to do so.'

Children's thinking about the motives of genetic and gestational parents they do not know will change with their developing ability to take the point of view of another person. Yet even when they become accomplished at anticipating what people they actually know would think or do in everyday circumstances, putting themselves in the shoes of strangers in unfamiliar situations will continue to challenge their understanding. Because they also have difficulty with ambiguity and ambivalence well into adolescence and beyond, it may be difficult to comprehend the panoply of viewpoints and circumstances that impelled anonymous but important people in their lives to make the choices they did. Perhaps the most parents can do to help is to introduce nuance and ambiguity into youngsters' more black and white judgments. The goal is to help the child develop as benevolent an image as is <u>honestly</u> possible of all the people who went about creating him.

Who Am I Anyway?

As they move into adolescence, children's interest in their origins operates in the service of identity development. Their question now is "<u>What does it mean about me</u> that I came into the world via an atypical route?" In thinking about how the special circumstances of their conception and birth affect children's thoughts and feelings about themselves, the particular technical assist involved will shape both what it will mean and how significant a part of their autobiographies it will become.

We can expect that children born from *in vitro* fertilization using their parents' reproductive cells will give relatively little weight to how they were conceived. Because they know all their parents, there is no more than the usual mystery about how nature joins with nurture to create the people they are and will become. There are no unknowns in the equation to pique their curiosity or inspire fantasies, romantic or forbidding, about who a missing genetic parent might be and what they themselves may have inherited from an unknown source.

Children born from surrogates who were gestational mothers only occupy a middle ground in this arena. They can be expected to be curious about the woman with whom they shared a unique biological intimacy. Although she may be a significant figure in their lives, it is the fact that they were in prenatal childcare, as it were, rather than who she is as a person that will address their questions about their own identities. A very vital part of their nurture, she is, at most, minimally involved in determining their nature.

It is the children born from collaborative reproduction using unknown donor gametes who, because they do not know both of their genetic parents, will face some of the questions about identity that confront children who were adopted. As they grow older, and especially as they approach adolescence, the task of building a stable, cohesive identity is challenged by what—and whom—they don't know. Like children who enter their families through adoption, they may think about who is their real mother or father, and, as in adoptive families, parents will want to talk with them about what it is that makes a parent real, offering both/and solutions to either/or questions. (See the next chapter for a fuller discussion of how to do this.)

Their quest for knowledge about the missing genetic parent is part of their search for a sense of self that integrates personality, temperament, talents, and interests. Unlike the adopted child, these children will usually have a history of being intimately connected to one of their genetic parents, skewing identification in favor of the known biological parent. How much interest a child shows in her genetic origins will vary from individual to individual. It helps when information is available, which a child may access or not, depending on interest. As with adoption, some but not all children born from donor gametes may choose to search for or meet an unknown genetic parent. Whether or not they are well-received at the end of the search, the grown children of sperm donors who have done so tend to report relief at filling in the missing parts of their history.

Children wonder, too, about having siblings they do not know. Most ovum donors and gestational mothers have children prior to collaborating in building families for others, and the number of possible children of a frequent sperm donor is staggering. Children may scan each new social group they encounter, asking themselves whether a brother or sister might be one of those present. Here again children's concerns mirror questions in the larger debate about ethical guidelines in reproductive technology. The public health interest in children's right to know who is a halfsibling—to avoid genetic inbreeding—is another compelling argument towards greater openness.

In thinking about how not knowing a genetic parent affects who they know themselves to be, the key difference between children born from donor insemination or ovum transfer and those who were adopted lies in having one parent who is also a source of their biological inheritance and one who is not. How the family has handled the genetic imbalance, whether it has amplified or diminished parental attachment to and identification with the child, will determine how much of an issue this becomes for the child as she addresses the question "Who am I?" by comparing and contrasting how she is like or unlike each parent.

Although it is somewhat different from when a couple decide to start a family together, experience with stepfamilies in which the remarriage occurs during the child's infancy has some bearing here. Children who know that Daddy or Mommy was not part of their prenatal history are not necessarily less attached to stepparents who have been part of their lives for as long as they can remember than they are to parents.

The greatest challenge for families formed by these means is to create a sense of equal psychological relatedness between the child and each of his parents, even though only one of them contributed genetically to his creation. It is vital that the adults maintain a commitment to deal with each other directly about differences between them in feeling empowered and responsible as parents rather than involve their child in their conflicts.

The imbalance may be more marked in children born from donor insemination. While ovum transfer, too, involves not being the genetic parent of one's child, mothers who have experienced pregnancy and birth may have a more visceral sense of connection to the child to whom they give birth than do nongenetic fathers. While not immune to feeling like less of a "real" parent than their partners, mothers in this circumstance may find that their biological history with the child offsets the genetic imbalance.

Care must be taken to avoid attributing too much significance to the differing genetic ties. For example, a mother who thinks of her husband as not sharing childcare equally may tell herself that this is so because donor semen was used to conceive—while in nearly every other house on the block moms must look to other factors to explain to themselves why they are shouldering more than fifty percent of the responsibilities for children who live with both genetic parents.

Both parents—the one who is also a genetic parent and the one who is not—need to have the kinds of conversations described in the next chapter about what makes a parent "real." It is especially important that the genetic parent talk to the child about how the decision to use collaborative reproduction to start a family was made by the parents together and that they are equally committed as parents. To say to the child, "Your dad is every bit as much your dad as I am your mom, this family is a joint venture" is important prevention against destructive coalitions within the family. To do so in no way precludes discussion of what it means to derive half of one's genes from another source.

Probably the best help parents can provide their children in psychologically integrating their prenatal histories is to work through any lingering ambivalence about infertility and how it was resolved. Ideally, parents will have worked out any lingering doubts, both for themselves as individuals and as a couple, before conception. In the real world, however, ambivalence and insecurity are not so easily dispensed with. Checking in on tender subjects from time to time to make sure their sensitivity is diminishing, taking steps, even seeking professional help, if soreness persists, can be essential to family happiness as children's development churns old issues to the surface.

The most important factor in children's psychological adjustment is how parents feel about how they formed a family. A parent who can discuss these issues matter-of-factly and without defensiveness, who is open to a child's questions about key figures in her conception and birth, will foster the child's positive self-regard. The story of "how you came into the world" need not be problem-free, but, if children are to feel good about themselves, it must be one that can be talked about freely without upsetting parents.

[1] I have just begun to interview children conceived through alternative means as part of a planned larger study, which is why there are fewer anecdotes in this chapter. So far, most of the parents who've volunteered their children to be interviewed are either single mothers or homosexual couples.

[2] The discussion in the stepfamily chapter about how to talk about halfsiblings may be helpful, although the circumstances are, of course, very different.

[*] See earlier chapters for a discussion of how to explain these words and concepts.

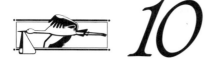

10
Talking with Children about Adoption

"My father's a dentist, my mother's a teacher, and I'm a dopted." Boy, 5.*

For the more than 50,000 children adopted each year, conception and birth are only the beginning of the story of how people form families. Adoptive parents are usually told to use the word *adoption* early, to lovingly relate the story of their own adoption to toddlers and preschoolers, to honor the contribution of the children's birthfamilies and culture, and to be open to children's questions and feelings about being adopted. Recent works have questioned this conventional wisdom, challenging the idea that young children can really understand these early teachings and highlighting the emotional obstacles for adoptive parents and their children in implementing these directives.

Like sex education, helping children understand adoption cannot be done in the "let's sit down and say everything there is to say and get it over with" mode. In *Being Adopted: the Lifelong Search for Self*, Brodzinsky, Schecter, and Henig, draw the parallel:

"As recently as a generation ago, being adopted seemed no different from being born into the family that raised you. We used to think that parents simply chose and received a perfect baby, told her at the age of three or four that she was adopted, and then went on to live a family life that looked just like Ozzie and Harriet's. Being told about adoption, went the thinking of the 1950s, was like being told about sex: the subject was raised carefully and appropriately, at the right stage in the child's development, and then it never needed to be raised again."

And, as with sex, parents' experience and further investigation shows that adults overestimate children's understanding of what they've been told and underestimate the need for continuing dialogue over the child's growing up years.

Early discussion of adoption is valuable even when and if children don't understand much about what the word means. Creating an atmosphere of openness and conveying how much they were and are wanted, being responsive to their questions, are all important parts of establishing a relationship of trust, so that children can take later concerns or confusion to their parents for help and support. It will take time, however, before children comprehend that adoption is permanent and before they can make sense of the web of circumstances that lead to adoptive families.

In a study designed very much like the one that formed the basis for the earlier chapters of this book, David Brodzinsky, Leslie Singer and Anne Braff explored children's thinking about adoption: what it means to be adopted, why some parents adopt children and other parents "make" children they do not raise. In questioning children about how and why families are formed by adoption, they found that there were clear and systematic changes in children's thinking as they develop. Very young children use adoption language before they have any idea of what the words mean and only gradually acquire the concepts that allow them to fully understand the concept of adoption. Their work underlines the need for a strategy of talking with children about adoption similar to that I've been discussing in conversations with children about the sex and birth.

"What does it mean to be a parent?" Brodzinsky and his colleagues asked 100 children aged four to thirteen, from both adoptive and nonadoptive families. "Suppose two people want to become parents—a mommy and a daddy—what do they do? Is there any way of becoming a parent besides 'making' a baby?" Later questions directly addressed adoption, including: "Let's suppose that a man and a woman wanted a baby and they decided to adopt one. What does that mean? What do they have to do? Why do you think they would want to? Is that child theirs forever? Where do you think the child would come from? What are the reasons that children are placed for adoption?"

The following discussion of the stages Brodzinsky and his colleagues formulated to describe how children's thinking about adoption develops is based on their analysis of the children's responses. Although the children I spoke with were slightly younger (3 to 12 versus 4 to 13), I will be describing their stages as they compare to the sequence of children's thinking about sex and birth, from Geographers to Putting It All Together, so that parents can integrate talking about human origins with discussing family origins.

Level One[1]: Parroting Adoption Language

Like the Geographers in Chapter Three, young children thinking about adoption have fewer questions than adults might imagine. For one thing, very young children have very different concepts of what a family is than do older children and adults.[2] People who live with you are your family, irrespective of the particulars of kinship or legalities. Family roles, like mommy, daddy, brother, and sister, are children's terms for adults and children, male or female. *Brother* is the name for young boy: there is no requirement that a youngster have a sibling in order to be a brother. And *mommies* and *daddies* get to have those titles when either they or their children decide to call them by those names. Remember the children in chapter three who explained that all grownups are mommies and daddies, whether or not they have children, and that parents get to be mommies and daddies simply by growing up and wanting children.

Because very young children assume that they themselves and all babies have always existed, they feel the need to account only for their whereabouts before coming to live with their families. The idea of getting a baby from another mother is not as remarkable to a two-to-four year old as it will later appear, nor is it something they see as necessarily requiring explanation. Alexandra, a nonadopted three-year-old (see chapter three) described her baby brother as having been in "someone else's tummy" and exiting from that someone else's vagina before being in her mommy's tummy, and Penny explained that a baby was passed from friend to friend like a gift before finally being given to the mommy. When children's ideas of all human origins take this form, adoption is not seen as very different than being born into the family they live with.

It is no surprise, therefore, that Brodzinsky and colleagues found that at the first stage of thinking about adoption, most preschoolers exhibit no understanding of adoption. Their responses are so idiosyncratic as to be unscorable. Even when they have been informed about being adopted themselves and use the word to refer to themselves, they frequently do not make any distinctions between birth and adoption as ways of forming a family. Nor do they understand how adoption takes place or the motives of either birth or adoptive parents.

How can they, when most children spontaneously explain that their parents got to be their mommy and daddy because either child or parents wanted each other? Here again, there are few distinctions between adopted and nonadopted children. It is not only hearing "the chosen baby" story, but children's own sense of magical omnipotence that leads many preschoolers to think of themselves as choosing or being chosen by the adults who are their parents. Again, the Geographers in my study, all nonadopted, regularly come up with statements like "because l like this mommy or "because I wanted to have a daddy and he gets me" or "because she wanted to be my mommy."

This similarity in children's thinking about adoption and birth as ways of entering a family is why negative feelings about being adopted are rare among preschoolers adopted as infants. The first sense of loss is likely to be a sense of having missed out on being in "mommy's tummy," a wish for a greater connection with the adoptive mother. "But I want to be in your belly," one two-and-a-half-year-old told her mommy, while another child, just past three, complained "I so sad, Mommy. I so sad I didn't grow in your uterus."*** Watkins and Fisher (*Talking with Young Children About Adoption*, Yale University Press) try to dispel parents' worries that joining in unrealistic play "gives it the stamp of permanent truth." The child who wants to play at growing inside mommy's body "may be trying to express her experience of or need for intimacy with you. Once she is allowed imaginal experience, the play moves on."

Talking with Children

In talking with your toddlers and preschoolers about adoption, remember that the objective is not to impart a lot of information. At best, they will only parrot your words with little understanding of what they mean. Like most children whose thinking is precausal, their interest is in where babies are before they come to live with their families, and learning the place they come from will satisfy their curiosity. Relating the story of their adoption with warmth and love, emphasizing how happy their arrival has made you (but not necessarily sharing the deep sadness of infertility), is the most important ingredient in the communication. They absorb the emotional message, even if they cannot grasp the intricacies of the concepts involved. In talking to two- and three-year-olds about adoption, parents need to be mindful that it is the feelings that underlie the story that their child will retain. While it is important to be responsive to any questions they may ask, detailed explanations will now be beyond their grasp. The goal of early teaching about adoption is to create an open, nondefensive atmosphere that establishes parents as trusted resources for later questions and concerns.

Level Two:"If Grandma's your birthmother, who's your adoptive mother?"** (3 1/2 year-old girl)

Children are now more responsive to questions about adoption. Like the Manufacturers in Chapter Four, they are beginning to grapple with the concepts of causality and identity. They now try to talk about the hows and whys of adoption and birth, but fail to differentiate between the two, which mingle and are fused in their attempts at explanation. They may either believe that all children are born to one set of parents and then go to live with another mommy and daddy or equate being born with being adopted.

Brodzinsky and his colleagues give several examples of how these ideas run together in the children's minds:

Alan,* at five and a half, said "Adoption means you go to try to get a baby, and if you can't, you can't." Asked where the baby comes from, he replied "From your vagina or your tummy." Whose vagina? "The baby's mommy." Is the baby adopted? "Yes... cause the mommy has it now. It came out of her." He went on to assent that all babies are adopted and declared that he didn't know if there was another way of becoming a parent.

Adopted preschoolers, like their nonadopted peers, confuse adoption and birth and generalize from their own experience. A five-year-old girl played at coming out of mom's skirt yelling "I'm adopted now," while a four-year-old asked, "Everyone's adopted, right?"*

Jenna,* at four, answered her interviewer this way:

Interviewer: Tell me, what does it mean to be adopted? What is adoption?

Jenna: It's like when you are small and you come home from the hopsital.

Int.: Tell me more. Exactly what happens in adoption?

Jenna: The doctor takes the baby out of the mommy and then they take the baby home.

Int.: Who takes the baby home?

Jenna: The mommy and daddy... First the mommy pushes the baby out of her and then she takes it home...The daddy takes it, too.

Int.: And what's that called?

Jenna: What you asked....adoption."

Andrew, also four, when interviewed for the Brodzinsky study, was able to describe the transfer of the baby from one "lady" to another:

Interviewer: What I want to ask you about is adoption. Have you heard the word before?

Andrew: Sure, I'm adopted.

Int: What does that mean? What's adoption mean?

Andrew: Well mommy told me that when I was a baby I came out of another lady... she made me. After I was born, my mommy and daddy came and got me and took me home.

Int: So first you came out of one lady and then you went home with another lady, your mommy... and of course your daddy too.

Andrew: Yep. That's how it happens.

Int: Is there any other way that grown-ups can become parents besides adopting a child?

Andrew: What do you mean?

Int.: How do grown-ups become parents? How do they become a mommy or daddy?

Andrew: They get a child... adopt him.

Int: Is there any other way of becoming a mommy or daddy?

Andrew: [Shakes head no.]

Int.: Do all kids come to their families after they are adopted?

Andrew: Yep... That's the way they do it.

For him, it is the only, the universal way people form families. Not distinguishing between adoption and birth, these youngsters have no knowledge of what adoption agencies are and do. They do, however, have some ideas about the motives underlying adoption. Wanting to care for and love a child, a desire to choose a particular type of child, wanting to increase family size, not being able to "make their own baby" and wanting to avoid pregnancy and birth problems were the most frequently mentioned reasons for adopting cited by younger children. Perhaps the hardest part of the adoption story for children to make sense of is how and why birthparents come to make placement plans. "Why would a woman who grew a baby give that baby away?," asked one four-year-old, "Why would she give me up?"** Because they see themselves at the center of their social worlds, young children's attempts to understand place-

ment look first at themselves, taking responsibility for both welcome
and unwelcome events. A four-and-a-half year old boy, for example,
who asked "Why didn't my real mom want me?" was asked by his
adoptive mother what he thought the reason was; he replied "I think
she didn't like me," while another child of the same age wondered
if he was placed for adoption because he was a bad baby or because
his birthfather was a bad father.**

When it comes to reasons why birthparents place children for
adoption, the four-to-seven year olds interviewed in the Brodzinsky
study were equally likely to mention not liking the child or thinking
the child is bad as they are to think of more parent-centered factors,
such as the financial and work problems—being too poor or too
busy or already having too many children—that make caring for
another child too hard.

How the child gets from one set of parents to another leaves
plenty of room for misunderstanding. For example, one five-year-old
told her mother "If it hadn't been for you, I would be with my real
mother" Her solution to the puzzle of why someone who grew a
baby would not then raise the child was to assume the child must
have been stolen: "You came and took me away."***

At this level, children are not entirely confident that adoption is
forever. This is not just a matter of not understanding that contracts
are legally binding. Young children's notions of who is family are
subject to the ups and downs of love and anger. In a study of children's concepts of family by David Pederson and Rhonda Gilby,
kindergarteners seemed to doubt that people originally thought
of as a family would continue to be one if its members did not love
each other. So, too, researchers Wynn and Brumberger found that
love was an essential element in defining family; for example, many
children declared that a father who moved out of the children's home
would continue to be a father, but only if he still loved the children.
When thinking about family is so tied to how people feel at the time,
it is not surprising that children might question what would happen
if birthparents, or adoptive parents, changed their minds about
placement, as when one four-year-old worried aloud that his birthfather might try to find him and take him away.

Talking with Children at Level Two

These are the children who are beginning to think through the adoption process but are not at all clear about how adoption differs from joining a family through birth. The question of whether and when to correct their misunderstandings is a delicate one: while it is important not to give false information, it is not necessary to correct every misunderstanding. How you respond to their versions of the adoption story might best be decided by the emotional weight of the inevitable distortions. "Original" ideas about their adoption need to be responded to one way if they give the child pleasure and another if they are a source of distress.

Nearly every child this age will say something like "I wish I grew in your tummy/uterus." Children whose play confuses birth and adoption, for example, may be expressing more than an immaturity in thinking. The two-, three- and four-year-olds who talk about wanting to have grown inside their adoptive mother's body are letting her know of their love; their wish is a symbol of the closeness they feel or want to feel. Telling the child who says "I was in your tummy" "No you weren't" misses the point, which is about relationship not origins. When the child has heard his adoption story before, your first response might be to say "You would like to have grown in my uterus" and give your child a chance to talk about his thoughts and fantasies about what that means to him. Some of the time you might remind him of his adoption day and having had a birthmother, but what is probably more on the mark is to tell him how much you love him and how you can't imagine feeling closer to him were he to have been born from you. Adoption educator Pat Johnston found that all three of her children responded well to being told "You know, honey, I wish you had grown in my uterus, too. That would have been very special. But since you didn't, I'm so glad I'm your mommy and you're my girl/boy now! I love you."

When the misunderstanding leaves them feeling bad about themselves or inappropriately angry at you or their birthparents, it is more important to "set things straight," but not before you understand what it is they do believe at the time. Some of the misunderstandings—thinking the adoption occurred because there was something wrong with them, that their birthparents were wrong for placing them, or that their adoptive parents have kidnapped them—are among those that need to be addressed.

Because it is "awfully hard" for children to know the array of circumstances that make birthparents unable to parent a child, they frequently assume that they were somehow to blame. When a child voices this belief, perhaps concluding that her birthmommy "didn't like me," you might continue:

Parent: It's so hard to understand why a woman who grew a baby could let someone else be the baby's mommy. Do you think it's because she didn't like you?

Child: Yes, if she liked me, she would have kept me.

Parent: If she had had a chance to get to know you, like I have, I'm sure she would have loved you very much, like I do. But she decided to have you adopted before you were even born—before she ever saw you. So I think we need to think together about what might be some other reasons why birthmothers can't always have their babies grow up with them.

While it is easy for children to imagine they were unwanted by their birthmothers, research tells us that women who plan adoption for babies often wish that they had been able to keep the children with them, think of them often, and maintain a lifelong affection and curiosity about a child not seen since birth. Caution should be taken, however, to avoid the other extreme of telling children "Your birthmother placed you for adoption because she loved you." You don't want children to feel that loving children leads to placing them, creating fears that their adoptive parents might follow suit. The goal here is to make it clear that while loving isn't what leads to placing, the two can coexist.

In addition to disabusing children of the idea that they were personally rejected, emphasizing that the adoption decision is usually made before the baby is born also protects against an image of the adoptive parents as predators, as when a five-year-old girl told her mother "If it hadn't been for you, I would be with my real mother...You came and took me away."** She needs to know that the decision that she would be adopted was made before the question of who her adoptive parents were to be was answered.

In giving adopted children the security that adoption is forever, current thinking is to avoid the image of "the chosen baby," first because it is often inaccurate in domestic infant adoptions: frequently it is the adoptive parents who are chosen for the child, rather than the child who is singled out by the parents who will raise him. But an even more important reason to avoid talking about the child as chosen is the insecurity it may give rise to, for what is chosen can also be unchosen. Brodzinsky and colleagues recount an anecdote from a woman whose adoption story included her parents walking among the cribs of an orphanage and being drawn to her because she smiled at them; her childhood was haunted by the concern about what would have befallen her had she not chanced to smile at that moment. And a man who'd been told by his parents that they had been shown two six-month-old boys and had chosen him as the "happier" of the two later found it difficult to let others know when he was sad.

Level Three: "'Cause that's the way it is when you're adopted.'"*

As they near five or six, children are beginning to be able to make classifications, to place objects in size places, and to more clearly differentiate between adoption and birth as alternative paths to parenthood. Brodzinsky and colleagues describe them now as accepting adoptive family relationships as permanent without understanding why. "At best they rely on a sense of faith ('my mother told me') or notions of possession ('the child belongs to the other parents now') to justify the permanent nature of the parent-child relationship". At seven, Emma, for example, says "Adoption means coming out of your first parents and then going to live with your second parents. The first ones are the ones who made you and the other people are your parents always. They have to take care of you and everything."* But asked why adoption is for always, a slightly younger girl could only insist "Cause that's the way it is when you're adopted... my mommy said so."

Recognizing that everyone enters the world in the same way, but that most children become members of the families into which they are born, children are now somewhat less positive about being adopted than they were earlier, when they considered adoptees as better off then their peers—brighter, happier, more popular, and more self-confident. Increased knowledge brings with it more expressed concerns, but Brodzinsky cautions parents against misinterpreting a child's raising difficult questions as reflecting underlying adjustment problems. Rather it is part of a normal process of their working through what it means to be adopted.

One thing it involves is recognizing that being adopted means having two different sets of parents. As mentioned earlier, children's earliest sense of loss in learning of the existence of a birthmother is usually to wish that they had grown inside the mother they know and love. Now that they can reliably make distinctions between parents and birthparents, they grapple with how to make sense—both intellectually and emotionally—of what they have come to know is not a typical situation.

In recent decades, the rise of alternative family forms—single parent families, stepfamilies, and families headed by grandparents or gay and lesbian couples—has made being adopted somewhat less out-of-the-ordinary. Indeed, it may be seen by some children as an advantage to have more than two parents without first having to go through a divorce.

Children are increasingly curious about their birthparents in the early elementary grades. Much to the chagrin of their parents, sometimes the distinction between birth and adoptive parents gets expressed in terms of "real" or "fake," One six-and-a-half-year-old told her brother, who was also adopted, "You are not my real brother. You are my fake brother. We are adopted. I was born from a lady in Georgia who really loved me a lot and she took care of me for a month and I was her Georgia peach. Then she gave me to Mom and Dad who adopted me and they are my fake parents. And we are a fake family."***

Questions from agemates about their "real" mother or father may prompt this way of framing the issue of how to reconcile having two sets of parents when most of their peers have only one. It is important that parents not take this as a personal rejection. Even said in anger, it is more likely an expression of momentary emotion than a dismissal of the parent-child bond. For example, one mother who had just angered her adopted daughter, then seven, recalls the following conversation:

Annie: You won't get a birthday card from my birthmother. Ellen only sends birthday cards to me.

Mother: Yes, you're the only one in the family who gets cards from her.

Annie: Ellen is my real mother.

Mother: Ellen is your real mother?

When Annie answered "yes," her mother found herself getting angry that her long-standing devotion was being so readily dismissed. "Then who am I?" she asked, only to melt when the answer came back "You're only Mommy."

Watkins and Fisher report one four-year-old explaining adoption to a friend: "The way I see adoption is like this. Somebody has the baby but can't keep the baby and goes 'Wah, wah, wah. Goodbye, Baby,' and somebody who can't get a baby in their tummy says, 'Oh great, a baby. Goody, goody, goody. Hello, Baby.' You know, somebody wins and somebody loses." In the next few years, thinking through the wins and losses raises some thorny questions.

How and why people place babies for adoption and others decide to adopt and raise those children is a topic to which children have begun to devote considerable thought. Asked why people might choose to adopt, six- and seven-year-olds spontaneously mention adults' desires to increase family size or choose a specific type of child, their infertility, and wanting to love and care for a child who would then provide companionship. Some believe that adults may prefer to adopt to avoid the hard work of infant care or the discomfort of pregnancy or birth.*

When the same children were asked to select the three best reasons for adopting from among several others, they most frequently chose reasons focusing on adult needs: "parents want to give love to a child" (67%), "parents want to have someone to love them" (33%), and "to remember them after they die" (36%). Somewhat fewer chose child-centered reasons: "Parents want to give a child a good home" (27%) and "parents feel sorry for the child who needs to be adopted(22%)". "Parents can't make their own baby" was selected by only six percent of this age group.*

The motives of birthparents in choosing adoption for children are harder still to understand, for many reasons. First, the source of information about the reasons for placement is often the adoptive parents, rather than the birthparent who actually made the decision. As such the explanation is based on indirect, at least somewhat inferential accounts. In addition, emotional considerations heavily influence what families are comfortable telling children about their birthparents. Most important, they want the children to think well of themselves, to dissuade them of any idea that they were "given away" because they were unloveable or bad. Nor do they want the children to feel that in adopting, the parent took advantage of the birthmother, as with the child mentioned above who thought of her parents as having taken her away from a birthmother who would have otherwise raised her.

Because they know more about the process of adoption, and are beginning to consider that all along the way there are unrealized possibilities, they become more concerned about mechanics, and what happens at "the waiting place," or the role of the adoption agency in placement. They may ask about things that could go wrong in the transition from birthparent to adoptive parents, like one almost seven-year-old boy quoted by Watkins and Fisher: "What if you or Dad hadn't been there when I came out of the lady I was born from?" When asked what he thought would have happened, he replied "They would have killed me," surprising his mother by remaining cheerful throughout this conversation. It is this lack of social knowledge that can lead to incorrect and even frightening interpretations of adoption, which should usually be seen as intellectual immaturity rather than psychopathology.

Talking to Level Three Children

Children at the third level in Brodzinsky's series of stages in understanding adoption, most of whom will range from four to eight years old, already clearly differentiate between adoption and birth as the means of entering a family. At this level they accept the permanence of adoption on faith and authority—parents have told them adoption is forever, but they don't understand how or why. The intellectual challenge for them now is to integrate the idea of having two sets of parents and to sort out the nuts and bolts of the adoption process, looking at how things work and what might have happened differently that would have dramatically altered their situations.

Parents can best help children think through these complex and challenging concepts by first looking at their own feelings and fantasies about their child's birthparents. Watkins and Fisher emphasize the importance of knowing what it is you really feel in order not to muddy the waters for the child who is seeking to understand herself better by exploring her biological origins. Only when parents are clear about their own unfinished emotional business can they thoughtfully plan what they would like to say to their child without having a hidden agenda.

Adoptive parents would prefer that children not think of the birthparents as the "real" parents. While it is certainly a valid point that what makes parents "real" is parenting, the day-to-day love and nurturing, care and responsibility for children, it is important not simply to override them when they fall into using this terminology, which is common among children. Often the best strategy is to make a shift in word usage without drawing attention or making a big deal about it. If the child asks about his "real mother", you might respond "Well, what I know about your birthmother is...." Remember the alternative to "real mother" isn't always "fake mother": it might be "mommy", as with seven-year-old Annie, quoted above. And it is not always adoptive parents who are relegated to 'unreal' status by children in this age group. One seven-year-old asked by a friend when he would look for his real mother, countered with "Richard, you don't understand. This is my real mother."***

When a child repeatedly refers to her birthparents as her "real" mother or father, however, and seems to be troubled as to whether she has a solid claim on the affections and attentions on the mother or father who actually parent her, you may want to talk about what makes a parent real:

Parent: When you talk about your birthmother as your "real mother," I wonder if it's hard to figure out how to think about having two mothers, a birthmother and a mommy?

Child: Yeah, most kids just have one. And when I say I'm adopted, kids ask me about my real mother.

Parent: It is sort of confusing, when things are different for you than for some of your friends. But let's think of all the things that "real" mothers do. Can you think of some?

Child: They grow babies that come out of their bodies.

Parent: Yes, so one way of being a real mother is to be pregnant and give birth. Can you think of other things real mothers do?

Child: Well, take care of babies, and make their lunches and their Halloween costumes, and work for money to buy them things.

Parent: Yes, so your birthmother is a real mother because she gave birth to you, and I'm your real mother because I do all the other things real mothers do.

Child: Can I have two real mothers?

Parent: You can have a birthmother and a mommy, and both can be real. Neither one of us is a doll or a puppet or a storybook character or something that's not real.

An eight-year-old boy quoted by Watkins and Fisher illustrates how children at this level of understanding can begin to coordinate having two sets of parents in a win-win way of thinking. After telling his Mom how much he loved both her and his Dad, he asked her "Is it better to have adopted me or given birth to me?" Asked what he thinks, he replied "I think it is just different." His mother then went on to tell him that she cannot imagine being any closer to him than if she had given birth to him, and he agreed that he feels the same way, "Me neither, I want you for my mother."

The idea of being a "chosen" baby or child continues to have a variable impact. On the one hand, a child may maintain that "being adopted is better because you're chosen," as with one seven-year-old whose adoption story went like this: "There was this lady, my biological mother. She was too young and too poor to be a mom, so when I came out of her vagina, my parents were waiting for me, and it was the happiest day of their lives."** On the other, an eight-year-old who asked his Mom if she had chosen him was relieved to learn that it was his birthmother who had chosen his adoptive parents: "That's good 'cuz if you buy something in the store and choose it, you can return it."** As they grapple with the motives behind both adoptive parents' and birthparents' choices and actions, they tend to become less sure, rather than more sure, that adoption is irreversible and the whimsy behind many of their own choices makes being "chosen" an insubstantial basis for the security they need.

Earlier I talked about the importance of dispelling younger children's ideas that they were placed because something was wrong with them. Four to seven-year-olds, report Brodzinsky and associates, focus on negative child characteristics in describing motives for placing a child for adoption, as well as the financial and other problems that might prevent a birthparent from taking care of the child. As they get older and more savvy about adoption, these latter reasons are emphasized and the idea that they were bad or otherwise undesirable recedes. Nonetheless parents are sometimes devastated to hear an eight-year-old son comment that his birthmother planned an adoption "because my ears stick out and I'm ugly" or a nine-year-old daughter state that her birthmother didn't elect to parent her because she was deaf, although her disability was undiagnosed when the adoption transpired. Helping them understand that it is the birthparent's life circumstances, rather than the attractiveness or behavior of the child, is still the focus of parent-child discussion of why children are placed for adoption. For now, most children accept the most frequently given explanation, of birthmothers "too young and too poor" or without family support as answers to this question, which emerges as still more puzzling in the years to come.

Level Four—Questioning Permanence

As children become firmly established in what Piaget describes as concrete operational thought, their understanding of family shifts away from defining family as those who share a roof, with biological connections not a necessary part of the relationship. By about seven or eight, children recognize that families are usually defined in terms of blood relationships. Knowing that they do not have a biological tie with their parents and that they have parents, grandparents, and maybe brothers and sisters elsewhere raises the issue of their status as family members.

Ironically, greater intellectual maturity complicates their understanding of and feelings about adoption. According to Brodzinsky and his colleagues, at this level, which may begin as early as seven and may range to as late as eleven, children clearly differentiate between adoption and birth but are more unsure than they were earlier about the permanence of the adoptive parent-child relationship. "Biological parents are seen as having the potential for reclaiming guardianship over the child at some future but unspecified time," they write in describing this level. The following excerpt from their interview of a seven-and-a-half-year-old girl depicts the child's dilemma:

Interviewer: Once the parents adopt the baby is it theirs forever?

Sara: I think so... unless maybe the other parents want it back.

Int.:   Could they get the baby back if they wanted?

Sara: Maybe, but they would have to want it back very much.

Int.:   Tell me more about that.

Sara: The baby's parents—the ones who adopted him— wouldn't want to give him back.

Int.:   What do you think would happen?

Sara: I think his real parents might get him back if they wanted him... maybe they have more money now and can take care of him better.

At about age eight or nine, children asked why people choose to adopt most frequently mention infertility, which remains at the top of the list for older children as well. Increasing family size, choosing a specific type of child, and the desire to care for and love a child were other frequently mentioned reasons for adopting. In the next phase of the Brodzinsky study, where children were asked to select the "best reasons" from among an array of motives for adopting, the eight- and nine-year-olds ranked wanting to give love to a child(65%) and wanting to give the child a good home (48%) or help the child grow up(30%) highest. Wanting someone to love them (25%), feeling sorry for the child who needs to be adopted (25%), and wanting someone to remember them after they die (15%) were seen as somewhat less compelling.

What most engages them at this point is the flip side of the adoption coin: the motives for placing a child for adoption. Because family is now usually defined by legal and genetic ties, rather than love and household membership, children want to know more about their birthparents. For the first time, developing the capacity for logical thought, deductive reasoning, and the ability to take the point of view of another lead them to seriously consider the circumstances surrounding their origins, to comprehend that being "chosen" means first having been "relinquished" and to consider the choices not taken by birthparents. According to Brodzinsky, much of the child's fantasy life between eight and eleven is focused on the possibility that birthparents might reclaim the child or disrupt the life of the adoptive family. As Michael, nine, put it "It's the master question of my life. Why did she give me away?" In struggling to understand complex situations and ways of thinking and behaving, they can be very judgmental of all the key participants.

Like younger children who think first of their own failings or defects as reasons why they might have been "given away," some children at this level also blame themselves. Melissa, at eight, opined, "Maybe I cried too much or didn't eat right, or something. I keep thinking that I did something wrong, like it was my fault, "* and Annie, at seven, repeatedly asked whether she had been placed because of her deafness, which was undiagnosed at the time of her adoption at ten months. More frequently, they now can separate out the circumstances that led to placement from their own value. Nine-year-old Virginia, for example, showed that she had absorbed her mother's earlier teachings. While she still was curious why her birthparents had "planted the seed" if they were unable to parent, she was clear that "she didn't give me away. She had a baby. She gave birth to me, but she didn't give me up."**

Their anger is now directed at others. Principal targets may be birthparents, as children reject those who they feel may have rejected them first. Drew, at seven, talked angrily of his birthparents: "I would punch them or drown them if I could. They stink... they didn't want me and I don't care 'cause they just stink."* And Megan, at ten, explicitly defended against feeling bad about herself: "I hate them for what they did. They didn't care enough to keep me. They just gave me away, like I was ugly or something."*

Not that they are immune to empathy with birthparents. The dilemma is how to resolve anger at feeling rejected while, at the same, wanting very much to feel love and admiration toward the birthparents whose worth reflects on their own sense of self-worth. One solution is to split the anger and the empathy, so that birthmothers remain in a positive light and birthfathers are blamed for the circumstances that led to placement. One seven-year-old quoted by Watkins and Fisher, remarked "You know it is not a nice thing for a man to give a woman a seed if she can't be a good mother yet... I've been trying to think this out in my head." While another child of the same age quoted by Brodzinsky and colleagues declared. "My dad is a jerk... he left my mom by herself."

When they were younger, the information that a birthmother was a teenager at the time was enough to satisfy their curiosity about why she wasn't able to raise them. Most middle class children see the teenagers in their community as more suited to babysitting than mothering. Now as they become more savvy about the larger world, they become aware that many pregnant teenagers elect to parent their babies, and they think long and hard as to which young mothers make the "right" choice.

Being young and poor suggests other remedies as alternatives to placement to children at this level. Perhaps there should have been more social supports available to young birthmothers, as nine-year-old Carla suggested: "If she didn't know how to be a mommy, then someone should have taught her. She should have gone to school to learn, then it wouldn't have happened."* Or the birthmother should have done more to help herself, as Monica, at eight, maintained: "If she didn't have enough money to be able to keep me, why didn't she get a job?"*

Nor are the parents they know and love exempt from criticism as they rethink the adoption process. The usual adoption story includes a birthmother who was "too young and/or too poor" to be a mommy, a reason that may now strain their evolving sense of social justice. Thinking of themselves as stolen or bought may target even much beloved parents as the villains in the drama. Erika, for example, at nine protested: "It isn't fair that (my adoptive parents) could buy me just because they have more money. Kids should be with their real parents. I'm not a toy or something you just decide to buy."*

Perhaps the safest target for children's anger in thinking of themselves as in some way rejected is to blame the impersonal agents of the adoption process—"the adoption people," be they social workers, lawyers, or agencies. Will, at seven, commented about his birthparents: "I think they might miss me and maybe are looking for me. They lost me when I was little... The adoption people took me from them and gave me to Mommy and Daddy, 'cause they didn't have a baby. I'm mad they did that."* How much easier it is to direct negative feelings toward unknown strangers, mere factotums in the process, rather than the adoptive parents on whose care they depend, the birthparents in whom they see their biological heritage, or themselves.

Talking to Level Four Children

In talking with children immersed in these issues, the key tasks are to help them address the ambiguities in their history, provide emotional support and acceptance in the face of their newly surfaced ambivalence about adoption, and assist them in finding their way back to confidence in the permanence of the adoptive family.

In a world of glaring inequalities, it is not always easy to satisfy children's curiosity about the circumstances of being placed for adoption in a way that allows them to feel well-disposed to all the participants. Parents need to be mindful to present all participants in as favorable a light as is possible, without engaging in deception.

Because their thinking is still concrete, their judgments tend to be black or white. Parents can provide perspectives that are beyond their children's experience that help them to temper outright condemnation with a more empathic view of the adults involved. In responding to the child who decided it was "not a nice thing for a man to give a woman a seed if she can't be a good mother yet", a parent can first acknowledge the child's empathy for the birthmother:

Parent: It sounds like you have a lot of sympathy for the difficult choices your birthmother had to deal with.

Child: Yeah, my birthfather must be a jerk. Why did he plant the seed if he wasn't going to help her take care of me?

Parent: It doesn't feel fair that she had to take care of things by herself. But men and women sometimes have sexual intercourse just because it feels good, without planning to have a baby. Sometimes they forget to use birth control, and sometimes the things they use to make sure the sperm and the ovum don't get together don't work. Sometimes birthfathers are jerks who leave the birthmothers to handle everything themselves, but other times birthmothers and birthfathers decide together what to do if the woman gets pregnant when they aren't ready to take care of a baby.

While youth and poverty are frequently key factors in the decision to place, it is vital not to overdo economics as the principal motivator. While material circumstances figure heavily in most important life decisions, they are only a part of the story. To exaggerate their significance, assuming they are self explanatory, runs against both reality and children's emerging sense of social justice. Most impoverished people raise their offspring, and prevailing value systems decry commercializing human relationships.

To children like Erika, the nine-year-old who protested to her parents that they had bought her like a "toy or something," raising the injustice of people getting children because they had more money, a parent might respond:

Parent: You're right, it isn't fair that it's easier to take care of chil-
           dren when you're not poor. It's easier to do a lot of other
           things, too, when you don't have to struggle to pay the
           rent or put food on the table. But we don't know for sure
           how important not having enough money was in your
           birthmother's decision that she couldn't raise you the
           way she wanted you raised. With important decisions
           like that, there are usually more than one reason.

Because other people can only guess about how a birthmother
viewed her alternatives or what she weighed in making the decision
for adoption, many experts now advocate that a birthmother write a
letter to the child she places for adoption, expressing in her own
words what went into her making an adoption plan, that can be
given to the child at a time when he or she is old enough to understand the complexities of her circumstances.

Children's concern and curiosity about birthparents and their
ability to think through the implications of events may now combine
to shake their confidence in the permanence of adoption. At level
three, they asserted that adoption is forever without being able to
say why that is so, relying on the authority of parents without
understanding for themselves. Now they are not quite so sure.
As they concern themselves with the morality of adoption-related
choices, they recognize competing needs, rights, and privileges.

If a birthmother wanted her baby back badly enough, they may
reason, how can they be confident that the adoption will endure?
Newspaper and TV broadcasts about custody disputes between birthparents and adoptive parents, of which the Baby Jessica case in 1993
was perhaps the most visible example, may make an exceedingly
rare event seem less remote than it is in actuality. They may need
reassurance that the stability of their home lives is protected by law.

Sara, the child who said "I think his real parents might get him
back if they wanted him... maybe they have more money now and
can take care of him better," could be engaged in a conversation that
might go like this:

Parent: After a lot of time passes, birthparents might be better
           able to take care of a child. They might even wish they
           had a chance to take care of the baby they placed for

adoption, who's a bigger kid now. Do you think they could then get him back?

Child: If they wanted him enough, I guess they could.

Parent: It's sad to think that someone who made a difficult decision like that can't change their mind when their life changes. But let's think about what that would be like for everyone. What do you think that would be like for the child, if one day someone came along, the child's birthmother or birthfather, who that child had never met before, and said "OK, I'm ready to take good care of you now, come with me."

Child: That would be weird. I think he'd want to get to know them, see what they were like, but if he had a good home, and loved his mom and dad and was used to his life, he wouldn't want to go away with them for good, even if he was born from them.

Parent: I think so, too. Most kids have a lot of curiosity about their birthparents, but they also feel that their home is with the parents they've known all or most of their lives, who've taken care of them and love them very much. Also, what do you think his mom and dad would feel about his birthparents getting him back?

Child: They'd hate it. There might be a fight. Or a tug of war, with his mom and dad pulling him to live with them, and his birthparents saying "You can't have him, he's ours now."

Parent: It's not good for a kid to worry that parents will fight over him. That's why the laws about adoption say that you only have a little while, only a few days or weeks or months, to make the decision to place a child for adoption. The birthparents have to sign a paper saying that they are making an adoption plan for the child, and they've thought about it enough to promise they won't change their minds. And the parents who are adopting the child sign a paper that he is their child to love and to help to grow up. The court then says that the adoption is final. That means they can't change their minds anymore, so the child can know that nothing can take him away from the family home.

Child: That's good for the kid and his parents who adopted him, but it's not fair the other parents can't change their minds. Maybe they made a mistake they want to fix.

Parent: That's why there's another way of providing for children whose parents can't take care of them for a little while. It's called *foster placement*, and it's different than adoption. Sometimes when people are having a hard time taking care of their children, if they're sick or have no place to live or something, they ask for help. Their children go to live with another family, called a *foster family*, but those children continue to see their parents and they all know that the parents hope to be able to take care of the children again. Foster placement is supposed to be for a short time, but adoption is forever.

Changes in how they are thinking about adoption cannot help but affect children's emotional lives. As their problem-solving ability allows for far greater understanding of adoption, youngsters' positive feelings about being adopted tend to decline, as reflecting on what it all means leaves them feeling confused, odd or different. They may become more private about repeating the adoption story that used to bring such pleasure; now it may evoke sadness and a wish to pass for "normal" or "regular."

For adoptive parents, these can be the most difficult conversations you will have with your child about what it means to be adopted. It is hard to see see their pain in feeling different or their envy of nonadopted friends who they see as having an advantage they lack. Brodzinsky, Schechter, and Henig describe how even those adopted as newborns grieve for their lost families once they develop an internal mental representation of what has been lost. They do not, however, show the "shock, deep depression, uncontrollable crying or intense rage" of those placed after infancy. Those adopted as older children have lost very real early caregivers and the rupture of attachment between parent and child make the transition to adoption both distressing and more difficult to understand. Instead, the losses of children whose adoptive parents are their only known caretakers are more abstract, and they show their grief "through confusion, occasional sadness, social withdrawal, or periodic outbursts of frustration or anger." In their daily travels they may look at passersby, hoping to see in the faces of strangers clues to their own origins. Brodzinsky says that searching for clues to their biological heritage is universal among adopted children and adults, even if no official search for birthparents is undertaken.

What it is important to keep in mind is that children's urgent endeavor to explain their world and how it came into being is neither an indictment of you as a parent nor a sign that they are "disturbed." Rather, it is part of the developmental challenge of growing up in a particular life circumstance. It does not mean that you aren't "good enough" or that they are "messed up."

Remember that the decision to adopt is not unconflicted for most adults either. For families begun by adoption, there have been losses to mourn and then accept: not having a biological connection to one's child can be as psychologically nettlesome for parents as it can later be for the children who must come to terms with not having a genetic tie to their parents. You've had time to work through some of your ambivalence about adopting before they arrived, Watkins and Fisher remind parents, now it's your children's turn to work through their own ambivalence about being adopted.

They will need your patience and support. Being available to listen to their concerns without defensiveness or self-justification is probably most important. Their emotional ups and downs are normal and temporary. If you can accept whatever it is they are expressing, acknowledging and helping them to clarify their feelings, they will make peace with their life histories, accepting and cherishing their families of nurture.

It is especially helpful if parents in a confidential adoption can find their way clear to responding to children's desire to know their birthparents by remaining open to their seeking more information in adulthood. When, your child expresses a longing to know her birthparents, you might say:

Parent: I know how hard it is for you to be so curious about them. If you still want to meet them when you're eighteen, I'll help you look them up.

A later section on open adoptions will address the issues for children who know their birthparents in childhood.

Levels Five and Six: Adoption is Forever—Again

Understanding the permanence of adoption characterizes the final stages of thinking about adoption, which differ from each other principally in the nature of the explanation of why this is so.

At Level Five, children's descriptions of the adoptive relationship are characterized by a "quasi-legal sense of permanence. Specifically, they refer to 'signing papers', or invoke some authority such as a judge, lawyer, doctor, or social worker who in some vague way 'makes' the parent-child relationship permanent." Brodzinsky and colleagues cite as an example ten-year-old Amy, who said: "After the people have the baby for some time, maybe a year or two years, they go to court and see the judge... They talk to him and sign lots of papers ...(that) say that the baby is theirs forever. It's up to the judge though... he's the one who says if it's okay or not."

At Level Six, with the beginnings of what Piaget calls formal operations, youngsters' ability for abstract thought makes accessible the concept of legal contracts, defining rights and obligations and the idea of a social contract that forms the basis for communal life. Not until early or middle adolescence do youngsters make the step to understanding that the adoption relationship is permanent because the rights and responsibilities for the child have been legally transferred from the biological parents to the adoptive parents. In illustrating this final stage in their hierarchy of understanding adoption concepts, Brodzinsky and colleagues cite Jimmy, 13, who gives the following explanation for why adoption is irrevocable: "Well, they have it legally now. It's their baby and now they have to care for it... not the other people. It's their baby forever... unless for some reason they find out that the parents are not responsible and were incapable of handling the child or something like that. You know, like if there's a case of child abuse or something they might want to put the child in a new home. Otherwise though it's their baby... the other parents don't have any right to the child now." His attention to the possible grounds for reversal, abuse or neglect, reflects the "relatively sophisticated and abstract appreciation of adoption as a sociolegal form of substitute child care—one based on the priniciple of protecting the rights and welfare of the child" that most children achieve by early and middle adolescence."*

A new appreciation of the social context for adoption leads to giving more weight to the needs of the child in considering the motives why parents adopt. Older children and young adolescents still spontaneously give infertility and choosing a specific type of child as the most frequent reasons why people choose to adopt, but they are followed closely by concern for the child's welfare and empathy for his needs, and wanting to care for or give love to the child. When choosing among possible "best" motives for adopting, a desire to give love to a child heads the list, followed by wanting to give the child a good home, help her grow up or take care of her. Motives that focus more on adult needs—wanting to have someone who will love them or keep them company or remember them when they're dead—which were chosen more frequently by the younger children, are absent or near the bottom of the list for those at the last two levels, who are usually ten-years-old and up. It's important to note that Brodzinsky and colleagues report no differences between adopted and non-adopted children in how they understand why people choose to adopt.

With increasing age and intellectual maturity, children no longer focus on negative child characteristics in explaining why birthparents place children for adoption. While they still mention a lack of time to take good care of children, financial problems are weighted even more heavily in accounting for this decision. They begin to stress birthparents' immaturity or inability to handle the responsibility of parenthood, and to mention family conflict, nonmarital birth, and parental death as additional reasons for placement.

Talking with Older Children

Moving from a quasi-legal to a legal basis in understanding the permanence of adoptive family relationships is part of children's emerging appreciation of the social underpinnings of human society. When their thinking is no longer limited to the people, places, and things that can be seen, heard, or touched, they begin to think about their own thinking, critiquing earlier notions and tying up the loose ends in the tapestry of family origins. In moving to Level Five, quasi-legal explanations, they have rejected earlier solutions to why adoption is permanent. No longer are they willing to take on faith parental pronouncements; "that's just the way adoption works" or "my mommy told me" no longer suffice. They now see the need for explanation rather than mere assertion. The recourse to social agencies beyond the family seems to offer a backup that provides more security to the adoptive arrangement.

In part, the move to a legal basis depends on more capacity for abstraction: inquiry into the principles on which family life is based, such as a responsibility to care for the next generation, and the philosophical basis for the larger question of how societies are organized and serve human needs. In talking with a Level Five child, a parent can address what it is that gives the judge or the court or the agency or the papers signed the power to finalize the adoption, underscoring that the process of transferring rights and responsibilities for the child is based on principle not individual caprice. For example, with Amy, the ten-year-old quoted earlier who talked about signing papers and it being up to the judge to make the adoption okay, a parent might continue:

Parent: What gives the judge the right to make it okay?

Child: Because he works for the government?

Parent: Judges have the job of making sure people follow the law. The laws about adoption are designed to make sure that children can feel secure in their homes and to make clear who is responsible for taking care of them. If the adults were confused about who could make decisions for children, they might not agree and the children's needs wouldn't get met. So the law sets up a way for the birth-parents to sign papers saying they give the rights to raise the child to the adoptive parents, who sign papers saying they will accept the responsibility to give the child a good home. And from that point on, the law says that they must do what they said they'd do. That's why we have laws, to protect our rights and make sure we perform our responsibilities.

As they approach adolescence, children become more and more intrigued with the question "Who am I?" When they have been adopted into their families, the paths they explore in creating a cohesive identity have some additional byways. They begin to raise more questions about history and lineage—how their personalities and talents may resemble those of their birthparents. Because what they look like becomes more and more important as they become teenagers, they become more curious about whom they may look like. And they seek to fill out their histories without alienating beloved parents on whom they depend.

Ian, a ten-and-a-half-year-old quoted by Watkins and Fisher, first stated how happy he was that his birthmother had given him to his parents because he loved them so much, only to follow that up with a statement that startled his mom: "Okay, Mom, I know it's different for you. I really do. But this is how it is for me. You will never be fully mine. Because I did not come out of your body. Because I was not made from your egg and Daddy's sperm. That's how it is for me."** Happily, his mom could remember that just the week before Ian had joked about still wanting to marry her, so that she knew "that some piece of this failure to 'be his' came from the normal developmental crunch of separating from his mom". But she was also aware that another piece came from his having to come to terms with the difference of adoption, so she responded, "You're right. That really is not how it is for me. For me you are so close that I feel sometimes that I did give birth to you. But... I hear that it's different for you. It's hard, Ian, isn't it, being adopted?"

He then felt free to tell her how he had kept silent about being adopted upon hearing kids at camp talk about how glad they were that they hadn't been.

Having permission to talk about how adoption sometimes makes him feel sad or different freed Ian to talk about adoption openly and with little distress. Studying family history in school, he decided to do a double chart—one for his biological history and the other for his family history. And when his six-and-a-half-year-old sister talked about his being a "fake brother" and their being a "fake family", he looked to his mom with a "what are we going to do with her!" look, and began "No, Lizzie, let me explain all this to you...".** Having parental support for the reality of his having a history which preceded his entry into the family, he can embrace the companion reality of being a very real part of a very real family.

Being able to hold on to this "double" reality is a key developmental challenge for adopted children, but it is not all that different from the task that all children face. Freud talked about the "family romance" as a fantasy children develop in the face of parent-child conflict as a way to come to terms with both loving and hating their parents at the same time. According to this fantasy, children decide that their frustrating disciplinarians must not be their real parents, who could not be so hateful. Instead, they imagine that they have been foundlings, whose "real" parents are better than the ones they know—"real" parents who will rescue them from the brutes who insist they clean their rooms or do their homework. Freud traced the idealized fantasy parents to the child's internalized image of the parent he knew in early childhood: "The whole effort at replacing the real father by a superior one is only an expression of the child's longing for the happy, vanished days when his father seemed to him the noblest and strongest of men and his mother the dearest and loveliest of women. He is turning away from the father he knows today to the father in whom he believed in the earlier days of his childhood, and his phantasy is no more than the expression of a regret that those happy days are gone."

It is not until they are mature enough to understand ambivalence. usually beginning between ten and twelve, that nonadopted children fuse their internal images of the fantasized "other" parents with the often frustrating real parents, who they come to accept as neither all good nor all bad, but human beings with both strengths and limitations. Adopted children, for whom the fantasized-about other parents are a reality, will usually take longer to work through the family romance. Chafing against parental restrictions, like all adolescents, they have a harder time reassessing their idealizations of their birthparents, when, as is usually the case, they have no direct experience against which to measure their fantasies. The temptation to believe, like Denise, at fourteen, that "the blood relationship would make a difference...they could just be with me and they would know what I needed, not like my adoptive parents," can be compelling to the teenager who needs to distance herself from mom and dad in defining what her identity is to be.

Accepting ambivalence in your children, and in yourselves, can be enormously helpful to preteens and teens coming to terms with the ambiguity of their family histories. Adoption aside, there is much to be ambivalent about in contemporary family life. Ideas of what families are "supposed to be" rarely match the possibilities for families operating in drastically different circumstances and taking increasingly complex forms. Families formed by adoption are one of the many variants on family life, as single-parent families, stepfamilies, and families headed by grandparents or gay and lesbian couples grow in numbers. Like other families that do not fit the *Ozzie and Harriet* or *Father Knows Best* format of the modern nuclear family that had its heyday in the post World War II period, adoptive families often struggle with wanting to fit the nuclear mold.

Canadian sociologist H. David Kirk divides adoptive families into two types: those that acknowledge and accept how they differ from families formed by birth, and those who reject all differences from biological families, with whom they feel themselves to be identical in every way. The denial practiced by the rejection of differences group impede children's ability to integrate their dual heritage into a coherent identity and can lead to emotionally constricted and limited relationships.

But Brodzinsky and his colleagues have added a third category: insistence on differences, that is, those families who emphasize how different adoption makes them from other families and tend to blame normal family events on their being an adoptive family. Exaggerating those differences that do exist, like denying all differences, can create emotional turmoil and interfere with the creation of close, loving family relationships.

In *Yours, Mine, and Ours*, which looked at how families change when remarried parents have a child together, I wrote about how conflicts within stepfamilies can be too easily diverted to questions of the family type, with stepkin saying to one another "You wouldn't treat me like this if you were my real parent/child." Adoptive families, too, can fall prey to this too available detour that both obscures developmental issues and creates unnecessary and problematic distance between family members. Giving too much weight to adoption in understanding what is happening between parent and child can be tempting, but reducing complex relationships to simple questions of form necessarily distorts both reality and possibility.

Accepting differences without exaggerating them requires talking about how your adoptive family is different from birthfamilies and also how it is the same. It means being open to discuss your child's concerns without insisting that every problem is traceable back to her adoptive history. One mother who adopted her first child and gave birth to her second, recalled: "When Jim was little and he would cling to me and not want to let me go, I used to think it was because he was adopted, that somehow he remembered being placed and was afraid I'd abandon him, too, or that he was insecurely attached or something. Then when Paul got to be the same age, and did some of the same things, I realized that that's what kids do sometimes. But with Jim, I was always so ready to see any problem as connected to his having been adopted." The rough spots in the life of an adopted child and her family may have little or nothing to do with adoption.

The adoption story doesn't end on the day the child comes home with you, or on the day the court finalizes it. Rather, the adoption story is a continuing theme, part of a serial on family life with daily installments, the meaning of which is constantly being viewed from new angles and is continually renegotiated.

Open Adoption

Open adoptions, in which the birthmother is both known to the adoptive family and is in continuing contact with them, were unthinkable during much of this century in the United States. Sealing adoption records first began in 1917 and did not become the norm until the 1940s, by which time social service personnel gained the power to enforce secrecy, in startling contrast to adoption practices throughout the world. This trend toward secrecy has been reversed in recent years, with an increase in open adoptions and a great deal of public discussion of adults adopted as children who later search for their birthparents.

What is meant by "open" adoption varies: At one end of a continuum, the adoptive parents and birthmother may know each other's first names and have arranged a means of getting in contact when the child reaches adulthood. Moving along the continuum, they may exchange photos at birthday or holiday times, have sporadic or regular visits, with the birthmother having the kind of contact with the child that a noncustodial parent might following a divorce. At the end of the spectrum, a birthmother may become a part of the extended family network of the adopting parents.

Because open adoption is relatively new, we cannot fully understand how it affects children—how they will manage multiple attachments, how they will make sense of who is related to whom and how among the people they know as family. As all families become more varied, however, having more than two parents is less unusual than it might have been earlier. Current projections, for example, are that by the year 2000, half of all the families in the United States will be stepfamilies. Children in open adoptions who know their birthparents share with their playmates the experience of having "extra" parents, but they are spared the pain of having gone through a parental divorce.

In talking to children about adoption, their knowing their birthparent, by name, by photo, or in person, fills in some of the blanks in the adoption story. Instead of talking about "your birth-mother" or "the lady", a parent can talk about "Ellen", who becomes more of a real person. Having more information may diminish the amount of time and energy that might otherwise be devoted to fantasies about who the birthparents might be. On the other hand, more knowledge can also prompt more questions, such as "how come Ellen didn't have Sally adopted?" when changed circumstances lead a birthmother to raise an older or younger half-sibling herself.

Annie, whose dialogue with her mother about Ellen being her "real mother," while Jeanne was "only Mommy," met her birthmother when she was seven. In Annie's letters to Ellen, Jeanne read an underlying subtext: Annie wrote "Dear Ellen, I'm six now, and it's time for my teeth to fall out" and between the lines Jeanne read, "Do you want to know me?" Anticipating the meeting her parents arranged during a family vacation, Annie wondered aloud whether to call Ellen "Mom," but when told she could decide for herself, she settled on 'Ellen." After the meeting, Annie was "incredibly relieved," according to her mother: "She used to agonize, and that helped her to come to peace with having been placed for adoption, although it's hard for her that she has a younger halfsister whom Ellen is raising. But Annie has a good deal, and I think she knows it."

Openness may answer questions, but it can also lead to disappointments if birthparents evince too little interest or to confusion if birthparents have not resolved lingering ambivalence about the adoption decision. There are as many possibilities as there are varying circumstances—familial, cultural, economic, and psychological. Knowing who birthparents are changes the child's experience of being adopted in some ways we can anticipate and others about which we can only guess. The stepfamily chapter may provide useful information.

Cross Cultural Adoptions

Years ago, agencies went to great lengths in "matching" children to their adoptive families. The guiding philosophy of the times was to make adoption as invisible as possible. Placing children in homes that reflected their physical, ethnic, and even religious heritage would allow the families to "pass" into the mainstream.

There continues to be controversy about interracial adoptions. The National Association of Black Social Workers has taken the position that African-American children not be placed in white homes, and the Indian Child Welfare Act mandates that children of Native American heritage be placed only with Native parents unless the Tribe consents. Nonetheless, more and more adoptions, whether domestic or international, involve children and parents whose ethnic heritages differ. The special challenges of interethnic adoptive families is first to help children feel fully enfranchised as family members, despite differences in appearance, and later to help them to integrate a sense of self that includes the cultures of both their biological and their psychological families.

For children noticeably dissimilar to their parents, physical differences in appearance mean that adoption is more a fact to be reckoned with on a daily basis than when it is not so apparent to strangers, friends, and the child herself that hers is an adoptive family. Casual acquaintances may insensitively inquire as to her origins, marking the child and the family as different. Playmates may ask "How can that be your mom? She doesn't look like you." Children will need your help in understanding that looking different doesn't mean not belonging.

Three-year-olds, intent on locating themselves in the social world, frequently look around and list who's male and who's female, who's a child and who's a grownup, among the people in a room. Sex and size are the two most important characteristics they focus on in organizing who's who. At first, physical characteristics are seen as randomly distributed. When my son was about three, for example, he asked me why none of the people in our "little family" had brown skin (as contrasted with "our big family", which included not only the usual array of grandparents, aunts, uncles, and cousins, but his halfbrothers' mothers and their kin, among whom were Native American cousins). But it is not long before children begin to recognize that in most families the range of hues is narrower than when there has been an international or interracial adoption. They compare their features to siblings, as well as parents, and they may be acutely aware that they are "the only one in the family who looks like me."

Children as young as three comment on the differences, usually expressing a preference for similarity. Watkins and Fisher quote a three-year-old who told her parents "Take off my skin, Daddy... Take off my hands, Mom, I want yours" and another, six months older, who has a play character tell her mother "Maya is sad... because she wants a mommy with brown skin, not skin like yours." She then suggests her mother paint her skin "and that if it rains God could help them keep the paint on," but later tells her "You can be my mommy forever and ever, anyway." When children still believe that a boy could be a girl if he wants to be, it is even less obvious that some aspects of physical appearance are unalterable. "Someday," an almost four-year-old suggests to her mother, "you should have skin on your hands my color."**

"There's my birthmother," they may call out whenever they see a stranger who resembles them or, less sure, they may ask "Is that my birthfather?" Like the children who say that a boat floats because it's red, confusing the relative effect of two attributes, an adopted Salvadoran child, for example, may assume that all Salvadoran children are adopted. As they become more familiar with other intercultural families, they can begin to recognize that "sometimes children from China have parents who don't look like them," as one Hispanic four-year-old in an Anglo family remarked upon seeing two Korean children with Caucasian parents.** This theme can be developed by parents, who can ask children to first consider what it is that makes a family. Most children under seven will focus on sharing love and a household as defining family, providing a basis for talking about how when people who love each other and live together have formed their families through adoption, the parents and children need not look like one another.

Probably the more complex challenge for children in intercultural adoptive families is to find a way to integrate their multicultural heritage. Physical appearance is not just a matter of genotype or aesthetics: different physical attributes have varying cultural meanings. Knowing as much as possible about the culture of their birthparents will both help children deal with how they are perceived in social settings outside the family and help them feel good about themselves.

Parents who make sure to include people of their child's ethnic heritage in their own social circles will boost the child's self-confidence. Feeling "one-of-a kind" raises the question: what does it mean when my parents say they love me, but don't seem to know anyone else who is like me? Nor can children feel proud of a heritage about which they know little and which marks them as apart from everyone who is important to them. Watkins and Fisher report a seven-year-old girl, adopted from Korea by a Caucasian family, who had previously tried to conceal her background, but returned from a Korean culture camp proud of her cultural heritage. Returning to school, she brought Korean objects to share with her classmates in the weekly "show and tell."

"Am I Indian?...Tell me about those Indians...," an eight-year-old asked his parents, "Those people were very smart...like me." Asking more questions about his birthparents, he announced he was going to tell his teacher "I'm Indian and I'm Greek...She's been wanting to know." In school projects that explore family history, it may feel "dumb" to make flags or family trees that chart only the adoptive parents' heritage. A more satisfying solution may be to make "four flags, one for each parent, birth and adoptive," taking ownership of all aspects of his identity.**

* I am deepy indebted to David Brodzinsky and his colleagues, including Leslie M. Singer, Anne Braff Brodzinsky, Dianne Schechter, Marshall D. Shechter, and Robin Marantz Henig. from whose important research on children's thinking about adoption I have relied heavily in writing this chapter. A single asterisk (*) following quotes indicates material from their work. Quotes from the very valuable work by Mary Watkins and Susan Fisher will be marked by a double asterisk. (**)

¹ Brodzinsky and colleagues have numbered their stages 0-5, For consistency's sake, in this book they will be renumbered 1-6.

² See Pederson and Gilby(1986), Beshars (1991), and Newman, Roberts and Syre (1993) for more on children's evolving concepts of family.

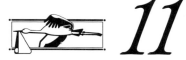

11

Making Sense of Stepfamilies

Talking about family building with children in families restructured by remarriage presents its own special set of challenges. Having weathered a series of family transitions, parental divorce or the death of a parent, children are faced with figuring out what this additional change will bring: What is a stepparent anyway, what will the relationship be between stepparent and stepchild, how will the child's relationships with his parent or parents be changed, and what if the new couple has a baby? How is the mutual child born to the remarried couple related to the children who danced, or cried, at their wedding?

At sixteen, Sean appeared in his school play and the family went out for ice cream afterwards to celebrate. His mother had flown in from her home 500 miles away. Because he had recruited Brian, then seven, to play a bit part, <u>his</u> mother, too, was present. When Sean's friends asked who everyone was, he told them: his Dad and Mom, his two halfbrothers and his first stepmother, and his second stepmother, who was then pregnant with his third halfbrother. "I felt weird," he later told his dad, even in their much divorced community. When David, Sean's youngest halfbrother, was, in his words, "four and five-sixes", he told his mother that for his fifth birthday he wanted another mommy, "I want you for a mommy and another mommy, a real mommy and a stepmommy." He was unresponsive to questions about why he wanted another Mommy, although he did know that a stepmother would be "either very nice or very mean." All three of his brothers had "another mommy," and he told his mother, "my first brain tells me I'll have a stepmommy when I get big."

Remarriage is increasingly a way in which people build families. Demographers' estimates for the early 1990s were that approximately one-third of all children would experience a parental divorce before reaching eighteen years of age; when separations that are not formalized by divorce were included, this figure jumped to two in five. More than half of these children will see the parent with whom they live remarry, so that one child in four will spend part of his childhood in a stepfamily. These figures do not include those children whose non-custodial parent remarries or those who acquire a stepparent through the marriage of a never-wed parent, the remarriage of a widowed parent, or when new partnerships are not formalized by marriage. Counting all the ways of forming stepfamilies, the numbers of children who will have a stepparent during some part of their growing up are immense.

In this chapter, the focus is on how children in stepfamilies make sense of the cast of characters in their complex families.[1] Wallerstein and Kelly (1980) have commented that children in remarried families are faced with an array of relatives that rivals a Russian novel in its complexity, but without the opportunity to refer to a diagram in the frontispiece for assistance in figuring out who's who. Nor are children the only ones having difficulty unraveling the tangles in the threads of stepfamily relationships. As a culture, our understanding of the kinship ties created by divorce and remarriage has not caught up with the demographic trends that will make stepfamilies the most numerous family form by the year 2000 (Furstenberg & Cherlin, 1991). Most people have no workable definitions of what a stepfamily is and how its members might be expected to behave towards one another.

Nonetheless, living in a stepfamily forces children to make sense of the family relationships of which they are a part. Children, the most naive stepfamily participants, that is, those with the least amount of cultural baggage from the world of nuclear families, are better able than adults to suspend preconceptions, attempting to understand a social situation as it is perceived and experienced. At the same time, the immaturity of their intellectual skills can make the task a challenging one, so that the child's efforts to understand stepfamily relationships will change with her developing cognitive abilities. Intellectual development, however, is not the whole story, how she feels about family members and how her own family is organized will color her thinking about who they are to her.

Can I Draw A Stegosaurus Now?

Two children within the same family will differ dramatically in how many questions they ask and at what age they begin to comment on how family members are related. Amber, for example, is described by her mother as "accepting the little realities of her social life as a state of nature," while her younger sister is a fountain of questions, asking about her halfsiblings' mother, "Who is she to me?" and "Why doesn't Daddy live with her anymore?"

A child shown photo albums from early on will come to identify his father's absent son as a brother, even though he has met him only once and their only contact is long-distance phone calls. Any steady state is more easily understood than erratic changes. And the more they know about the older children's whereabouts when they're gone, the less preoccupied they will be with their comings and goings. When a stepchild is back and forth between houses at frequent intervals, the mutual children who have been to the other home are well aware of where he is. Although they may cry when the older children go, there is no mystery when such departures are routine. Unlike adults, who have a set of expectations of family life that include all members sharing a household full time, children born into stepfamilies can accept such arrangements as "a fact of life."

Typical of preoperational thinkers, many of the younger children interviewed said they didn't know what a family was, although all could list the members of their own families. Those who would venture a definition said a family is "people," or "something a lot of people live in, a lot of people." According to a five-year-old it is "people living together," or, as a four-year-old put it "You love all together." Residence and caring continue to be the criteria children use throughout the preoperational period, moving on to definitions that primarily list family roles with the transition to concrete operations, e.g. "A husband and a wife, and two, usually two or three children." Concrete thinkers focus on conventions and rules for relatedness, both biological and legal. As they enter their teens their definitions become more philosophical, engaging issues of meaning and purpose.

Understanding what is meant by "step" relationships takes on a similar progression, but it is not universal. In families where the older child's other parent is out of the picture, this prefix may play no part in family life, and younger children may learn late, even in adulthood, that both parents did not produce an older sibling. Sometimes parents delay giving their mutual child information about an older child's parentage for fear of giving him a weapon that can be used against her. Leslie, for example, tells that she does not plan to tell her son Oliver that her older daughter, Denise, had another father "until he's much bigger" than four. "If it comes into conversation, of course, we'll talk about it, but I don't want to make any differences. If it were brought up, then it would be like 'Well, this is my Mum and Dad'. I would really hate that to come in. It would be like a power thing that would be easy to use." Others delay giving this information because they think the child is too young to understand, leading him to fantasize that their lives run on parallel tracks. In one such family, one mother described her son as echoing her stepdaughter's stories, assuming that all her relatives are also his: "After Barbara finishes her story about 'my grandmother this and my sisters this', Anthony will say, 'Well, my grandmother this and my sisters and brothers', making up a story just like hers."

More usually, however, children use the vocabulary before they can accurately construct its meaning. Step relationships may be seen as part of everyday family life, as when David, making a Play Doh™

family of worms, identified them as "the mommy, the daddy, the brother, the other brother, and the stepsister. But use of "step" vocabulary does not imply conceptual understanding. At two, David could verbalize that his mother is his brothers' stepmother. At three he was still asking:

David: Are you my stepmother?

Mother: No, I'm your mommy.

David: Then who's my stepmother?

Mother: You don't have a stepmother.

David: But I want a stepmother, too.

As he listened to this conversation, his older halfbrother Brian, then ten, shook his head incredulously. A later discussion between mother and son revealed that David, at four, still did not grasp what was meant by the terms that had been part of his vocabulary for two years.

David: Why does Brian have to go to Judyann's house?

Mother: She's his mommy, and she likes to have him live with her, too.

David: Brian has two mommies.

Mother: Judyann is Brian's mommy and I'm his stepmommy.

David: You mean she's his real mommy?

Mother: Yes.

David: You're joking.

When family members are defined perceptually, e.g. a sister is "a girl in your family" or a mother as "somebody who takes care of children," it is difficult for children to differentiate between mother and stepmother, sister and halfsister. For most of the three to six-year-olds, all mutual children, a stepparent is another parent, for example, Aileen, at four-and-a-half: "I don't know what a stepfather is, but it's another father. And Eva's a stepmother. Another mother." Or Amos, at four-and-a-half: "Jeremy has two dads. One is ours." There is a recognition of a difference, but no articulation of that difference. Owen at three-and-a-half, said of his brothers, "I don't know why they have their mom." At four-and-a-half, Ethan says a stepmother is "something kind of like a mother," but when asked what the difference was replied, "That's a hardie. Can I draw a stegosaurus now?" Aileen, more venturesome at the same age, suggested that her brother had two houses "Because fathers can't live together and mothers can't live together. There has to be one mother and one father, so the stepfather and the plain mother live here, and George's stepmother and real father live there." The first attempt at distinction usually involves this use of the word *real* as the antonym to *step*. So that a stepmother becomes "a mother that's not really your mother." (See the chapter on adoptions for additional discussion on what makes family members real.)

At first glance it may appear that the propensity of the younger children to begin their definitions of stepparents as supernumerary parents is the result of their being mutual children, the offspring of the current marriage, not stepchildren. Stepchildren are certainly more likely to make clear distinctions between a parent and a step-parent. Unfortunately no comparison could be made between step and mutual children of the same age. Because the families I inter-viewed had to have a mutual child who was at least three years old, and because the transition from divorce or bereavement through single parenthood to remarriage and another child usually takes a number of years, children in this age range are less likely to have both a stepparent and halfsibling.

But even stepchildren may first think of a stepparent as anoth-er parent. For the Geographers in Chapter Three, all women are mommies and all men are daddies. To get to be a parent, you have merely to eat your vegetables, brush your teeth and follow the other imperatives of childhood until you are grown up and, by definition, become a mommy or daddy. If any adult is a parent, a stepparent might then be conceptualized as "a daddy that's not really yours."

Asked to explain how their parents and siblings got to be members of their family, the smallest children attribute magical powers to wishing and wanting. Children frequently describe their parents as being their parents because "He wanted to be my daddy," which can be extended to explain the relationship with siblings, as when Erica, at four, insists that Nila "just came out born, and she wanted to be my sister, so when she grew up she was my sister." Who came out of whose "tummy" also figures prominently in their explanations of why older children have a different mother, while paternity is harder for them to account for. It is obvious to Erica that her halfsisters live elsewhere, and she claims she has never wondered why, "because they didn't come out of my mommy's tummy."

Another characteristic of this egocentric early stage is that the younger children are, from the age of three, able to tell how each family member is related to him or herself, but often have some difficulty in explaining how the others are related to each other. They cannot yet see relationships from another's perspective. It is as if *brother, sister, father* and *mother* are labels people have, more on the order of *Fred* and *Alice*, than a statement about the connection between them. Oren, at four, knows that Dan is his brother, but it is not at all clear what he understands that to mean, since he identifies his dad as Dan's "cousin," denying that he could be Dan's dad too, and says that this adult halfbrother has a father who lives "in the same house as he is." Erica, at four- and-a-half, identifies her mother as her halfsister's "friend," but later says that sister is her mother's "child," albeit in a different way than she herself is.

Like the preoperational child who can tell if there are more red beads than blue beads, but not if there are more red beads than wooden beads, these youngsters are not yet capable of keeping categories constant and look to nonessential clues of appearance or activity to make distinctions about relations. Often three- to five-year-olds will explain that their full siblings are related to them in a different way than their halfsiblings because one is bigger than the other. Four and a half year old Alana has a younger brother, Aaron, and an older halfbrother, Ken.

Me: How is Ken related to you?

Alana: Ken is my other brother.

Me: How did Ken get to be your brother?

Alana: He was born in my family."

Me: Is he your brother in the same way as Aaron or in a different way?

Alana: Different, because he's bigger than Aaron.

Me: Are there any other differences?

Alana: That Ken can do more things than Aaron.

Me: You told me that Aaron was related to you because
           he lives with you and that Ken doesn't live with you.
Alana: He's still my brother, and he doesn't live with me,
           because he has a different mom than mine."

Some of the fundamentals of step relationships can be grasped
relatively early. Eve, at six-and-a-half, could explain that her mother
is her halfbrother's stepmother "because they're my dad's children
and not my mom's children." And Ina, while unable, at five, to
distinguish in any way other than size between her older sister and
her teenage halfsister, at almost six could add another distinction:
"Pam is here half the time and at her mom's half the time." In these
middle years, both the step and mutual children start to explain
relationships in terms of history, often starting with an account of
the initial marriage, the offspring it produced, the divorce, remarriage and its offspring. For example, Enid, at nine, explained how
her father's older daughters are related to her by running down
the milestones that formed the family: "Her mom and my dad
were married, and they had Bonnie and Judith. And then they
got divorced, and my dad married my mom, and they had me and
Andy." At that point a stepparent is defined in terms of a network
of relationships, for example, Alissa at eight: "When somebody
already has a baby, and then they get divorced from that person,
and get married again, the new person that they marry is a stepmother or a stepfather."

At this level, which corresponds to the In-Betweens in Chapter
Five and the Reporters in Chapter Six, children are acquiring concrete
operations, and quantification and measurement of relationship
are an important part of their approach to figuring out relationships.
Beverly, for example, at seven-and-a-half, describes a stepfather as
"part of your family, but it's not your real father. He's part of your
father and your real father is all your father." Blood-relatedness is
often depicted quite concretely in terms of sharing blood, flesh, or
genes. Thus, a halfsibling may be described as "someone who has
half your blood and half someone else's blood," or, by a girl of ten,
"I just think of her as my sister. I mean flesh and blood, half of her
at least." "Step" is also interpreted very concretely as in "a step
removed from," so that Angela at seven-and-a-half defines a step-

mother as "a step away from who is your real mother," and Tamara at ten, describes her stepfather as "kind of like a step over" from a father. There were no systematic differences between stepchildren and mutual children in how those in this age range defined family relationships.

With the transition to formal operations, preteens and teens begin to give explanations of relationships that are multidimensional and well-reasoned. They can coordinate a network of relationships and take different points of view, so that relationships are seen as reciprocal and contingent on other relationships. They do not need to trace out the historical sequence of family events to give a coherent definition of a given relationship. Instead, they can "put it all together:" abstracting the essentials, integrating the impact of affection and social convention, without getting the various strands tangled. A halfsibling is now "someone born through your stepfather and mother or your stepmother and father," according to one twelve-year-old.

Understanding from the Heart

If a glass can be described as either half full or half empty, so can steprelatives be described as more like or more unlike blood relatives depending on how a child feels about them. A seven-year-old may begin her definition of a stepmother with "they're nice to you," while a nine- year-old who omitted her stepmother from the list of those in her family, when asked how they're related will say "I'm sort of not," going on to say that a stepmother is "another mother who didn't have you," defining by negation. Those children with basically positive feelings toward their stepparents tend to make distinctions while minimizing difference, like Carl, at sixteen, who says his stepfather is "the same thing (as his mom), at least for me, helps bring me up, helps raise me." In contrast Bert, also sixteen, says, "I think of her as a stepmom...I think there's always, no matter how hard you try, unless you don't like your mom, you have some resentments towards a stepmom."

Even children in the same family will have strikingly different definitions of a stepparent, based on the differences in their attachment to the parent who remarries, as when one sister defines a stepmother as "a woman who marries your father who is not related to you," while another, speaking of the same woman, calls her "a friend, a really good friend, and the mother of my sisters." And a daughter who remains loyal to the father who left the family may accept her stepmother, extending herself and reaching out to the older woman as a way of staying close to her father, identifying their child as her sister, while her brother, who was their mother's defender in the family drama, may deny any relatedness to either.

Paula, at eighteen, reflects the warmth achieved over the years, although not without struggle, of her relationship with her stepmother in her definition: "The woman my father met after being separated with my mom and fell in love with. Technically she's my stepmother because they got married, but she's also my stepmother in the sense that she mothers me." Whereas Brendan, at fifteen, cynically defines a stepfather as "someone that is married to your mother for the second time." He laughed, "or the third time, I guess, or fourth or fifth."

When a mutual child is asked what a stepparent is, she is talking about her own mommy or daddy, and her definitions generally reflect the greater empathy with the role based on their greater closeness. "I was going to say a second mother," explained Anita, at eighteen. "Who is not by birth your mother," she went on to elaborate, "but chooses to mother. She may not choose to, but has married your father, and is therefore stuck with that job."

Definitions of stepparents are especially loaded for stepchildren, because they call into play questions of loyalty. The same child may vary how he thinks of his relationship with a stepparent, giving differing accounts to others, even the stepparent himself. One day when Brian was seven, he angrily told his stepmother "You don't have sons, or stepsons, only friends," yet before the month was out he held her hand to his face and called her his "Annie Mommy". Even step-relationships that extend back to the child's infancy must be differentiated from the primary ones the child fears disavowing. Asked how she was related to her stepmother, fifteen-year-old Jillian struggled with how much a stepmother is the same as or different than a mother:

Jillian: She's married to my father, and she's given birth to my two halfbrothers and halfsister, and I've lived with her for thirteen years. She's like a second mother to me...Even when I say that, I don't really think of her as a mother. I guess I really do, and that's just me using that she's a stepmother against her... I've lived with her for a long time. She's just really another mother when I'm here. ...She's not really another mother. That's mean to my mother, but she's like a second mother."

More than any other family roles, mother and father tend to pull for exclusivity: it's okay to have more than one child, grandparent, aunt, or sister, while to think of more than one person as a mother, or as a father, smacks of treason.

If loyalty conflicts can color the way stepchildren define a stepparent, so too can rivalry serve as an emotional pollutant in their understanding of halfsibling relationships. Nancy, at nine-and-a-half, clearly distinguished between how related she felt to four-year-old Elaine and seven-month-old Abbot. After she had described Elaine as a "halfsister" which she defined as a "sister that's not really your sister," I asked her how she is related to Abbot:

Nancy: He was born, when he was born he just came my brother.

Me: Is he your brother in the same way as Elaine is your sister or in a different way?

Nancy: A different way. He's my real brother, he's not like my halfbrother or halfsister or something like that.

Me: What makes him your real brother when Elaine's your halfsister.

Nancy: I don't know.

Me: What do you think?

Nancy: I guess it's just like the age or something. Because after my Dad married her, she didn't have Elaine yet. So I guess when Abbot was born, then he would be my real brother.

Me: What makes Elaine a halfsister and Abbot a real brother if they have the same mother and father?

Nancy: My Dad married Janet, they had Elaine and then they had Abbot. I guess that just makes Abbot my real brother, because they had him after they were married.

Me: Was Elaine born before the marriage?

Nancy: No.

Me: Is Abbot your brother in the same way as or a different way than Brenda is your [older, full] sister?

Nancy: Just the same.

Me: Is Elaine your sister in the same way as or in a different way than Brenda is your sister?

Nancy: Brenda is my real sister and Elaine is my halfsister.

Elaine, whose birth when Nancy was five must have felt like more of a displacement than did the arrival of the infant brother who was born when she was nine, was in a category all her own: interloping halfsister.

Mutual children in stepfamilies also construct relationships differently, denying either difference or similarity, depending on the emotional loading and circumstances. Two extremes are represented by Orianne, the seven-year-old eldest mutual child in a family marked by some tension between her mother and adult halfbrother, and Alexander, twelve-and-a-half, the only mutual child in a step-family to which both his parents brought older children.

Orianne does not spontaneously include her adult halfbrother in her family, but when asked if anyone else was in her family, quickly adds, "My big brother."

Me: Is your mom related to your big brother?

Orianne: I'm not sure.

She goes further to deny the biological relationship between her father and his eldest son:

Orianne: He grew up with the same father, except he was a little different from a real brother, so he has a different mother.

Me: How did John get to be your brother?

Orianne: Because his father died, and my father had to marry again. So he married my big brother's mother, and so he became my brother.

Me: Is your father also John's father?

Orianne: Yes, but first he had a different father, but I don't know
           <u>anything</u> about that.

Twelve-and-a-half-year-old Alexander, on the other hand, goes
to great lengths to minimize distinctions in a family in which both
parents brought a child from a previous union. Speaking of his
father's relationship to his mother's daughter, he says:

Alexander: He's really like her whole father, but he's not really her
           father. I think he's starting to believe that and she's start-
           ing to believe that he is, and I can see why. They're so
           tight and their birthdays are only one day apart, so they
           can't be that far away from each other.... I wouldn't call
           it a stepfather-stepdaughter relationship, I'd call it a
           father-daughter relationship."

Me: What's the difference?

Alexander: In that kind of relationship, they're not understanding
           each other, getting into a lot of quarrels, not listening to
           each other. That would really be considered a family that
           has some step-relative, who really doesn't know how to
           take the place of a real father or mother."

Mutual children are less likely to make distinctions among
their siblings than are the older children whose consciousness of
being in a stepfamily is more acute. None of the children of remarriage that I interviewed spontaneously identified a halfsibling as
such until queried further about relationship, whereas several of
the stepchildren did so. The mutual child would often insist, like one
eighteen-year-old, "I never think of them as half anything. It's just
technically that's the relationship," or the thirteen-year- old who was
adamant that he considered his mother's older daughter "my full
sister." When differentiating degrees of relatedness, the mutual
child is more likely to counterpose "full" to "half" siblings, unlike
some of the children from earlier marriages for whom the distinction
is between "half" and "real". For these older children, a reference to
"my brother" or "my sister" that lacks a name or birth order qualifier, like "my younger brother," always refers to a full sibling.

Sixteen-year-old Larry, contrasting his thirteen-year-old brother Kevin from their three-year-old halfbrother, Owen, demonstrates how the children of both of one's parents are seen as more of a fact of life, whereas the mutual child is more of an optional addition to the family: "For me, my brother has always been my brother, so I don't really think about who he is. I just kind of accept him. I never thought about what it would be like without him, because he's always been there."

An example from the family that opened this chapter illustrates how a child feels more related to someone who has been related since birth: When Brian was seven and his stepmother was pregnant, he said that the baby would be his stepbrother. When she explained that her son would be his halfbrother, just like his then sixteen-year-old brother by his father's earlier marriage, Brian protested: "Sean's not my halfbrother. He's been my brother a long time."

While the emotional ties to half and stepsiblings are usually clearly differentiated, the language used to describe them remains confusing. Children use half- and step- almost interchangeably for quite some time, often continuing into adulthood. The youngest children maintain that there is no difference, and seven- and eight-year-olds say "it's kind of the same thing." In striving for consistency, children may insist that the their stepparent's baby must be their step-sibling. It takes cognitive maturity as well as emotional reconciliation with family realities to sort out why children born to a stepparent prior to remarriage are related to them in a different way than those who share a parent with them.

Mom's Child, Dad's Child

Whether the parent they share is a mother or a father is seen as a criterion of the strength of the tie to a halfsibling by children who are in primary custody with one parent. Beverly and Jenny, both seven, have a one-year-old halfsister Angie. Beverly lives with her mother and stepfather, who is Jenny's Dad. Jenny visits every other weekend.

Jenny, who shares a father with the baby, originally identifies baby Angie as her stepsister, then corrects it to halfsister.

Me: How is Beverly related to Angie?

Jenny: I guess it's just her sister.

Me: Is Beverly more related to Angie than you are?

Jenny: I guess it's almost the same.

Beverly, on the other hand, who shares a mother with the baby, originally identifies Angie as "my baby sister".

Me: How is Jenny related to Angie?

Beverly: That's her stepsister, and it's part of her sister, and it's the same thing. I'm kind of related that way to Angie...It's Jenny's sister too, it's her real sister, not her stepsister.

Her first impression is that Jenny is Angie's stepsister, because Jenny is Beverly's stepsister. Only when she deduces that they are equally related to their halfsister does she correct her initial formulation, so that the baby is the "real" sister of both girls.

One adult stepchild told of learning from her inner city schoolchildren that a father's children were stepsiblings and a mother's children just plain brothers and sisters, 'cause "You came out of the same stomach." Her own eleven-year-old halfsister echoed this approach to which is which when she told me, "Well, a stepsister is your father's daughter, and a halfsister is your mother's, but it might be vice-versa." This reasoning is echoed by nine-year-old Barbara, who contrasted her paternal halfbrother, with whom she lives full-time following the death of her mother, with her mother's other children.

Barbara: I have two sisters and a bigger brother, which are my real sisters and brother. Anthony's not actually my real brother, because Edith's my stepmother.

Me: What makes the older children your real brother and sisters?

Barbara: They were born to my real mom.

Me: So, you have the same mom and different dads?

Barbara: Yes.

Me: Why does having the same mom make someone more of a brother than having the same dad?

Barbara: He was born from somebody else, dads don't have babies.

Although she earlier said that dads were a necessary part of making babies, Barbara is very concrete in her thinking: seeing is believing, and paternity is still too abstract a concept to have equal weight with the more observable connection between mother and child.

But the sex of the parent is not the only, or perhaps even the primary, factor in these assertions of "mother right". None of the children in joint custody, including several who had both parents with additional children, felt that a mutual child was more of a brother or sister depending on whether it was their mother or their father who had more kids. Sharing a household, growing up together, more than anything else, is what makes children feel connected to one another. "We're related socially and emotionally," said Joanne, referring to the children of her father's remarriage, "because we partially grew up in the same family." In contrast, a woman whose relationship with her father remains a difficult one told me "I don't usually think of my family as including my dad's part of the family. If this were under any other circumstances, I would just draw my mom's part of the family".

When The Mutual Child Has Been Adopted

Although parents and children alike tend to stress the fact that a mutual child is related to all of them, creating enduring ties between people otherwise more tenuously connected, biological relatedness may not be as important to his centrality as equidistance to all stepfamily members. It can be just as important that the mutual child be linked genetically to nobody as to everybody. A mutual child who is adopted into a stepfamily as an infant occupies a similar position, representing the unity invoked by the remarriage, with many if not all of the dynamics common to yours, mine, and ours stepfamilies.

When Jack was eight, his father and stepmother adopted a baby boy. Jack, who lived more of the time with his mother, remained somewhat reserved with the baby, telling his stepmother that they weren't real brothers. He was startled to hear her say that the baby, Will, was just as related to Jack as he was to her, whom he clearly regarded as Will's mother.

What makes Jack and Will halfbrothers is not the presence or absence of a shared genetic heritage. They are halfbrothers because they have the same father and different mothers, and it is this network of relationships that lays the groundwork on which their own brotherhood will be built.

The Extended Stepfamily

One morning during breakfast with their uncle's family, Tonio, then thirteen, asked if Natty, Kate and Morghan were David's "stepcousins." Basing his reasoning on the common confusion of halfsibling for stepsibling, he explained: "I thought because he's my stepbrother he might be their stepcousin." His uncle reminded him that David is his halfbrother, and his mother went on to explain the kinship of cousins.

Stepmother: Cousins are only related on one side of the family. Since you're related to these cousins through your dad, not through your mom, and you and David have the same dad, David is related to Natty, Kate and Morghan exactly as you are.

Tonio: So would I have stepcousins?"

Stepmother: My brother's children are your stepcousins.

Tonio: Oh, Greg and Mark.

When we look beyond parents and stepparents and their children to the larger family network, relationships become still more complex. The paucity of relationship terms compounds the ambiguousness of any relatedness with a sibling's kin. Nor is there a social consensus about what constitutes relatedness in stepfamilies. It is no wonder, therefore, that for the child, figuring out whether her mother is related to the stepsister she acquired through her father's remarriage is no simple matter. And in response to questions, children struggle to put the pieces of the puzzle together in a way that feels internally consistent.

Essentially the solution to the question of who is related to whom is arrived at via one of two strategies. The first is to apply the selfsame criteria used by the child to define the family: household membership and propinquity. Children of remarriage using this approach recognize the distance between themselves and their half-siblings' relatives. In answering whether they are related to their halfsiblings' other parent a three-year-old will say, "No, 'cause she's not in our family" and a four-and-a-half year old will elaborate, "No, because she didn't live with me ever." At eight, a girl answered the same question by pointing to behavioral criteria, "I'm not related to Lili because I don't go to her house to spend time like Pamela does." When there is no contact between the mutual child and the extended family of the first marriage, the question is simplified: it is harder to conceive of being related to someone when, according to a seven-year-old, "I never even saw her."

But not all children are as exclusive in their concept of relatedness. Some of the children demonstrate a remarkably expansive definition of family. Greg, for instance, at seventeen, includes his mother's boyfriend's children, whom he has never met, in listing family members. Although he feels estranged from his former stepfather, he includes the older man's mother as "a real grandma, real family." Inclusiveness, as an approach to claims of kinship, stems either from affection or from striving for conceptual consistency.

Frequently, children present with a firm conviction that relatedness must be reciprocal: If my mommy is your stepmom, then your Mommy must be my stepmom. Even children who see themselves as not related to their halfsiblings' other parent may try to find a way of claiming kinship with the older child's other halfsiblings. At eight, Alissa knows she is not really related to Pamela's halfsister from her mother and stepfather's marriage, "but when we were younger, we used to call each other 'half-halfsisters'," she told me. Her younger sister, Ida, at five, in trying to figure out her own relationship to "Pamela's sister" labels her "my stepsister," even claiming Pamela's mother as her own "stepmom."

Me: What makes Jackie (her father's ex-wife) your stepmom?

Ida: She didn't have me.

Me: I didn't have you. Am I your stepmom, too?

Ida: (Laughing). No, she didn't have me, and I see her sometimes.

No matter how inclusive they are inclined to be, children have to draw the line somewhere. For example, Ike, at seven, claimed his mother's first husband as his stepdad, but of that man's new wife he said, "She's not related at all."

Children are slow to recognize time's arrow in their understanding of relatedness. Angela, at seven, reported that "I never met (her older halfsisters' mother), but I think she is sort of like my stepmother. But she really isn't, because I have a real mother right now. She's sort of my stepmother." Eleanor borrows from the kinship terminology for cousins in describing her older halfbrother's mother as her "stepmother once removed." And Amber, at eleven, speaking to the same issue, says that she and her halfsisters' mother aren't related "any more." When queried further, she says, "I guess she never was."

How and why people are related can be difficult to untangle even for children at the brink of formal relations. Witness this bright eleven-year-old, attempting to figure out if Yale, his mother's younger son, is related to his father's stepson:

Brent: Is he? Let's see... I'm related to my dad, but my dad isn't... When you marry, do you become relatives? I don't know. If now my stepmother is related to my dad, then he would be related, but if not, then he wouldn't be?"

Me: Is your dad related to Yale?

Brent: He has to be, because he's my brother and this is my dad. I don't know how it would be. I don't know what it would be called."

The idea here seems to be that two people who are both his biological relatives must be related to one another, but that one of

his relatives-by-marriage may not be related to another of his biological relatives if he is the only link.

One solution to the question of who's related to whom, used
even by children who are quite small, is to divide the concept of family into "our little family" and "our big family," "the four of us" or
the "seven of us," as a reference to stepsiblings who no longer live
at home. "Our big family" then becomes easily expandable to include
the other parent of the older children, as well as grandparents,
cousins, and other traditional members of extended families.

Constance Ahrons, in describing the two household family of
divorced parents and their children as the *binuclear family*, points
out the paucity of our vocabulary for describing the relationships
between individuals in the remarriage chain. So far, I have described
the cognitive developmental barriers to children's conceptualizing
stepfamily relationships, the impact of emotional factors, and the
structure of the family on their cognition. But when a culture lacks
words to describe so many of the relationships in the extended family of divorce and remarriage, conceptual handles for grasping these
socially meaningful categories are unavailable, for adults as well as
children.

There is no name for the relation of the present and former
spouses of the same person, no name for the relation between a
parent and his children's halfsiblings, no name for the relation
between children who are each the halfsibling of the same child.
And the vocabulary of kinship we do have is itself inadequate to
denote the relationships it does name: for example, stepmother is
used to describe any woman married to one's father, whether she
is seen once a year or every day, whether she has principal responsibility for raising a child or is a friendly occasional visitor, whether
the mother is in the picture or not.

Piaget, in describing the development of cognition, emphasizes
the role of experience. Those aspects of the environment with which
the child interacts most frequently and most actively are those which
are mastered earliest and with the greatest sophistication. When
environmental access is limited or, in the case of stepfamily kinship
categories, impoverished, assimilation of concepts is slowed. While
part of the difficulty for children in figuring out who is related to

whom in stepfamily relationship networks may be due to their slowness in understanding the time factor in this genealogy, it would be
a mistake to attribute this, or other holes in their conceptualizing,
exclusively to intellectual immaturity. Rather it reflects an arbitrary
assumption of our culture that the kin of the current marriage are
considered related to the progeny of the former, while the offspring
of the current union bear no relation to the kin of their older halfsiblings. Children's "mistakes" underline the slowness with which
social categories follow upon contemporary trends in American
kinship patterns. Lacking complete induction into what there is of
current social convention, those children who insist on a reciprocity
of relatedness with the kin of their kin may, like the little boy in
The Emperor's New Clothes, simply be reporting reality as they
perceive it: a kinship structure enlarged by divorce and remarriage
to create what has been called "the new extended family."

Talking With Children

Knowing that children will not fully understand the complexity
of stepfamily relationships is no reason to avoid talking with them
about matters that affect their daily lives. First, answering children's
questions honestly and clearly, matching the information given
to their ability to comprehend, lays the groundwork for a trusting
relationship between parent and child. Knowing that their questions
have been responded to honestly helps them to continue to ask
questions, trusting parents to help them sort out confusion and
dispel worry.

For confusion can lead to worry, as it did for the little boy
who thought that he would have to live half the time in another
house when he was bigger, like his brother whose joint custody
arrangement meant that they shared a home only half the time.
Knowing why the older boy left, that he had a daddy in another
house and they wanted to spend time together, could reassure him
that an arbitrary eviction was not on the way for him.

Confusion can arise, too, when children lack the words that
enable them to process differences they perceive, as when a young

girl senses that her father is different with her than with her sisters. When she is told that he is her stepfather, she has a way of thinking and talking about a host of observations that had theretofore been both unsettling and undeniable. When the discovery that a sibling is a halfsibling or a parent is a stepparent is made indirectly or by chance, the secretiveness involved gives rise to feelings that the family status of one or the other family member is something shameful.

What's a Stepparent?

Perhaps the most inclusive definition of a stepfamily refers to the unit formed when a parent of one or more children establishes a new partnership with another adult, whether through remarriage or by setting up a household. The early stages of stepfamily life involve a "getting to know you" period, during which time steprelatives experiment with who they are to one another.

It is essential to clearly differentiate stepparents from parents, in order to save children from the loyalty binds that make accepting a stepparent and eventual stepfamily integration more conflictual. Both parent and stepparent need to introduce the idea that a stepparent is <u>another</u> caring adult in the child's life, rather than a replacement for a parent, living or dead.

Child: When you marry Ellen, will she be my new mommy?

Parent: No, when we're married, Ellen will be your stepmother.

Child: What's a stepmother?

Parent: A stepmother is your father's new wife, and a new member of your family.

Child: Will I have two mommies?

Parent: No, your mommy will always be your mommy. But a stepmother does some of the things that a mother does. She can have fun with you, and helps to take care of you.

In talking with children about what a stepparent is there is no right answer. Being a stepparent means inhabiting an ambiguous role: who you are to the child will vary on how old he is when you enter the family, how much time you spend together, how much contact he has with both his parents, and how comfortable your partner is with sharing childrearing responsibilities. Within one household, a stepparent may have very different kinds of relationships with each of the children. A stepfather entering a family with three children, for example, might become almost a "second father" to the three-year-old, more of an "uncle" or "counselor" to a ten-year-old, and a "big brother" or "special adult friend" to a teenager.

While lack of role clarity is normal in stepfamilies, and clarification among family members can decrease conflict and improve relationships, there is virtual consensus that new stepparents go slow in being "parental" to their partner's children.

Toward this end, stepfamily experts agree that it is best not to require the child to call a stepparent *Mommy* or *Daddy*. Most advise allowing the child to take the lead in deciding what to call the stepparent, although it is also important that children use a different word for their stepparent than they do for the parent. For example, a child who wants to use a parental form of address for her stepfather might be encouraged to use *Papa* if she calls her father *Daddy*. Many families are comfortable using first names, while others will want some means of retaining generational courtesy, such as *Mama Jean* or *Daddy John*. When children have different ways of addressing mom and stepmom, dad and stepdad, the risk of setting off an explosion of possessiveness (if father heard stepfather referred to as *Daddy* or mother heard stepmother referred to as *Mommy*) is minimized, and children are freer to develop affectionate ties to their stepparents.

When There's a New Baby

When a remarried couple is expecting a child, they frequently hope that the baby will be a unifying force, legitimizing the family membership of a stepparent who is not also a parent or solidifying a sense of being one family among the children they already have. Children may be apprehensive, however, wondering how the new arrival might mean less time, less attention, and fewer material resources for them. In talking with children about the impending birth of a mutual child, it is important both to emphasize the connection between the child and her brother or sister-to-be and to allow her to be ambivalent about having to adjust to yet another family change.

Timing the announcement of a pregnancy is critical in stepfamilies. The expectant couple should be the ones to inform their children that they are going to have a baby, so that the children learns this from people who can convey the news with pleasure. It is equally important that their parent inform his or her ex-spouse about the pregnancy before the children have occasion to do so. In this way, the adults can deal directly with each other about any distress one may have in hearing the other is about to have another child, and the children are not exposed to the full force of any parental negativity on this score.

After saying "We're going to have a baby," parents can stress the forthcoming relation between the children by talking about "your brother or sister." Most stepfamilies in which the children have even intermittent contact do not add the half- qualifier in describing sibling relationships. Young children might be expected to think, very literally, of a halfbrother as the left side only of a boy or a halfsister as a girl from the waist up. Helping them to sort out exactly how they are related will take a number of conversations.

Frequently, children are told by the expectant parents that they will soon be having a new brother or sister, only to return from their other household with crushed spirits and the news that "My father says the baby isn't my brother, he's only my halfbrother."

A parent might respond:

Parent: How do you feel when you think of the baby as a half-brother instead of a brother?

Child: Not so good. Half a brother doesn't sound like it's as good as a real brother.

Parent: Well, a halfbrother is a whole person, and you can have fun with him, play with him, and grow up with him. You're brothers because you have the same mommy (or daddy), and because you can do all the things that brothers do together. The only thing that makes him a halfbrother is that you have different daddies (or mommies). Strictly speaking, we call two children halfbrothers or halfsisters if they have one parent who is the same and one who is different.

Especially if they have different mothers, children may refer to the baby as a stepbrother or stepsister. A stepmother might respond:

Child: When my stepsister is born, will she share my room?

Stepmother: When your sister is first born, she'll sleep in our room. Why do you call her your stepsister?

Child: Well, you're my stepmom, so your baby should be my stepsister.

Stepmother: I can see how that might seem to follow. But you and the baby have the same daddy, so you aren't stepsisters. If I had had a little girl, who had a different father than you do, before I married your dad, then that little girl would have been your stepsister. But because this baby is both mine and your daddy's, she'll be your halfsister— because you have one parent who is the same, and one who is different.

Parents can expect that how the children are related to one another will continue to be negotiated and renegotiated throughout their years of growing up. How close they will feel, how much like brothers and sisters they will consider themselves, will depend on a number of factors: the custody arrangements for the older children, whether they share a mother or a father, how their other parent feels about the stepfamily household, and how close they are in age. If they barely know each other and have little contact, their brother- or sisterhood will be an abstraction: either an irrelevancy or a hanger on which to drape their fantasies. When, however, they live together, day in and day out, collecting a storehouse of shared experiences, the consequences of their halfsiblinghood are diminished.

At a dinner at his cousin's house when he was five, David surprised his mother by stating, "I have three halfbrothers." On the way home, twelve-year-old Brian said something about having a "real brother," and David countered with "Brian's not in the real family." Their dad then insisted that both were part of the "real family" and both were "real brothers," but the matter was far from closed.

No sooner had they entered the door than David threw himself on the couch, sobbing inconsolably, "I only have halfbrothers." Told what David was crying about, Brian went in to say, "I'm your brother, David." When David had calmed down, his mother asked him how he heard about "halfbrothers," a new word at their house, despite all the talk about her being the older boy's stepmother.

David: (His cousin) Neil told me Billy is Neil's halfbrother, and
            I'm a only a halfbrother to Brian and Tonio and Sean.

Mother: Do you know what makes Brian your halfbrother?

David: Yes, because he was born from Judyann."

This gave them an opportunity to talk further about what makes two boys brothers.

Mother: Sharing the same parent or parents is only one of the
            things that makes you brothers. There's also living
            together, knowing each other from the time David was
            born, loving each other and fighting with each other,
            all the things that brothers do, and you can't get much
            realer than that.[2]

Such discussions will go on over the years, helping each boy sort out how family politics shape their brotherhood. As with anything else that children learn, there will be things that they understand now and complexities they will not be able to grasp until later. Yet to withhold all information until complete comprehension is possible deprives them of the opportunity to make things better between them now.

A final word on a frequent concern of stepfamily couples as they anticipate having a child together. Typically, a prospective parent who had no children before becoming a stepparent worries that her own child will follow the example of her stepchildren in calling her by her first name. Wanting to, finally, be somebody's mommy, the stepparent wants the older children to start calling her *Mommy* so that the baby will learn by imitation how to address her.

This approach is unsettling to the older children, setting a precedent for their needs being subordinated to the mutual child's.

Nor is it necessary to accomplish the goal. Children born into step-families can and do learn to call their parents *Mommy* and *Daddy* even if their older halfsiblings call them by other names. After all, children typically address their parents by different terms than the adults usually use in talking with each other.

This does not mean that the younger children won't test the limits. As a two-year-old, for example, David knew that he could always get his mother's attention with the following litany: "You're Sean's stepmother, you're Tonio's stepmother, you're Brian's step-mother, you're my stepmother." But if parents don't overreact to a child's verbal explorations, they will soon lose interest for him. Quietly telling the child that you want to be called *Daddy* or *Mommy*, and not responding to unwanted terms of address will usually be effective.

---

[1] For a more extensive discussion of stepfamily relationships and how families change when remarried parents have a child together see Bernstein (1990) Yours, Mine, and Ours.[T4]

[2] See the chapter on adoptions for an extended discussion of how to talk to children about what makes relatives "real."

Afterward

There is never just one way to organize a book. In thinking through how to integrate new material with old, it seemed best to deal first with children's evolving understanding of sex and birth, both as a universal part of the story of human origins and as a way of introducing a developmental perspective to how children make sense of the world in all its complexity. By introducing the subjects of stepfamilies, adoption and assisted reproductive technology, I hoped to be more inclusive of the increasing numbers of families formed in these ways. I suspect that some parents for whom these concerns are most pressing may have read through the early chapters impatiently, wondering when their special circumstances would be taken into account. I hope they find their persistance was rewarded in the end.

I would like now to encourage those who may have skipped over the last three chapters, thinking these did not apply to them, to reconsider. Even married couples who are their children's only parents will find their world increasingly populated by families for whom this is not the case. It is important that all families inform their children about the various ways that people create families. To neglect this part of teaching children about how parents get to be parents places an undue burden now on children whose beginnings are not typical, forcing them to make the difficult choice between educating their peers about family diversity or suffering in silence during discussions that leave them out. Later, it may foster psychological conflict in today's children whose own family and reproductive options in the future cannot be predicted.

When I married a man with three sons and then went on to have a first child who was my husband's fourth, I built on my early interest in children's understanding of sex and birth by investigating children's experience of stepfamilies. In thinking about how to talk with children in this edition about different ways that people build families, it seemed important to include ways of discussing the stepfamily relationships that demographers estimate will affect half of the people in the United States by the year 2000. In a culture still so influenced by the Brothers Grimm that *stepchild* remains a popular image for any person, organization or project that is not properly treated, supported or appreciated, stepfamily members struggle to feel like theirs are "good enough" families. "Normalizing" stepfamily life for all children, whether or not they are stepfamily members as children, will help to allow them to grow up to create effective, nurturing and enjoyable families, whatever their structure.

Children who were not adopted do not need to learn about adoption quite as early as those who are, but by the time they start school they will often have encountered playmates whose family story includes adoption, necessitating the introduction of those concepts. Openings for starting conversations with nonadopted children will occur when friends or family members adopt a child or make an adoption plan. Noticing when the word *adoption* occurs in the media, a parent can ask his child, "Do you know what that means?" The dialogue that follows can lay the groundwork for later discussions, which can be responsive to questions as they arise. Care should be taken to cultivate empathy if children demean the situation of the other child. Questions that invite the child to walk a mile in the shoes of the other, considering how she would want to be responded to under similar circumstances, can help to create positive, respectful attitudes toward others.

With children born through assisted reproductive technology, there is less consensus about how open to be, both with the children and in the community. While different medical interventions have different levels of social acceptance, each is stigmatized by some portion of the community. Other reasons for secrecy stem from unresolved ambiguities about the rights and responsibilities of each of the parents—social, gestational, and genetic. Writing on medical ethics, theologian Gordon R. Dunstan and sociologist Geoffrey D. Mitchell suggest that the question should not be "Should the child be told of his origin?" but rather "What social and legal adjustments must first be made, to make the telling safe?" In making public policy around these issues, perhaps the best criteria for the social arrangements that accompany reproductive innovations lies in the answer to the question, "Is this something that a child can learn about his origins without compromising his self-esteem?"

Making these subjects part of every child's education creates a social climate in which each child can take pride in herself and her family, mitigating the controversy that surrounds family diversity. "Family values" has become a catchword for decrying the ways that social change has redefined who gets to call themselves a family. Values about family are deeply felt. They are central to how we think about ourselves and our possibilities, and most people will want to pass on to their children their values about how family life should be. At the same time, the future of civil society demands that children learn family values in ways that discourage violence— be it physical or psychological—on those whose values differ.

However most parents disagree with the choices made by other adults, no child decides how she will be born, or to whom, and few have any say about who will raise them. All children deserve the opportunity to grow up feeling they are worthy of respect, without which they cannot learn to respect the rights of others. Whatever we teach our children about making choices about sexual behavior and family composition, we must also teach them not to judge other children by how they got to be in their families and who else is there.

Sources

Ahrons, Constance R. and Rodgers, Roy H. *Divorced Families: A Multidisciplinary Developmental View.* New York: W. W. Norton, 1987.

Ashmore, Richard D. and Brodzinsky, David M. (Eds.) *Thinking about the Family: Views of Parents and Children.* Hillsdale, NJ: Lawrence Erlbaum Associates, 1986.

Barbach, Lonnie Garfield. *For Yourself: the Fulfillment of Female Sexuality.* New York: Doubleday and Company, 1975.

Beilin, Harry and Pufall, Peter. (Eds.) *Piaget's Theory: Prospects and Possibilities.* Hillsdale, NJ: Lawrence Erlbaum Associates, 1992.

Bernstein, Anne C. *Unravelling the tangles: Children's understanding of stepfamily kinship.* In William Beer (Ed.), *Relative Strangers: Studies of Stepfamily Processes.* Totowa, NJ: Rowman & Littlefield, 1988.

Bernstein, Anne C. *Yours, Mine and Ours: How Families Change When Remarried Parents Have a Child Together.* New York: W. W. Norton, 1990.

Berntsein, Anne C. and Cowan, Philip A. (1975) "Children's Concepts of How People Get Babies," *Child Development*, 46, pp 77-91.

Beshers, Julie Gricar. "Strategies Children Use for the Cognitive Construction of Kinship." *Sociological Studies of Child Development*, Volume 4. (1991) JAI Press, Inc. pp. 137-151.

Bonnicksen, Andrea L. *In Vitro Fertilization: Building Policy from Laboratories to Legislatures.* New York: Columbia University Press, 1989.

Brodzinsky, David M., Singer, Leslie M. and Braff, Anne M. (1984) "Children's Understanding of Adoption," *Child Development*, 55. pp. 869-878.

Brodzinsky, David M., Schechter, Marshall D., and Brodzinsky, Arne Braff. "Children's Knowledge of Adoption: Developmental Changes and Implications for Adjustment," Chapter Eight in Ashmore, R.D. and Brodzinsky, D. M., *op. cit.*, 1986.

Brodzinsky, David M., Schechter, Marshall D., and Henig, Robin Marantz. *Being Adopted: The Lifelong Search for Self.* New York: Doubleday, 1992.

Chadwich, Ruth F. (Ed.) *Ethics, Reproduction and Genetic Control.* London and New York: Routledge, 1987.

Cooper, Susan L. and Glazer, Ellen S. *Beyond Infertility: The New Paths to Parenthood.* New York: Lexington Books, 1994.

Dunstan, G. R. "Social and Ethical Aspects," in Carter, C. O. (Ed.) *Developments in Human Reproduction and their Eugenic, Ethical Implications.* London: Academic Press, 1983.

Flavell, John H. *Cognitive Development.* Second Edition. Englewood Cliffs, NJ: Prentice-Hall, 1977.

Fraiberg, Selma H. *The Magic Years: Understanding and Handling the Problems of Early Childhood.* New York: Charles Scribner's Sons, 1959.

Freud, Sigmund. "On the Sexual Theories of Children." (1908) In Reiff, Philip (Ed.) *The Collected Papers of Sigmund Freud.* New York: Collier Books, 1963.

Furstenberg, Frank F., and Cherlin, Andrew J. *Divided Families: What Happens to Children When Parents Part*. Cambridge, MA: Harvard University Press, 1991.

Gadpaille, Warren J. *The Cycles of Sex*. New York: Charles Scribner's Sons, 1975.

Kagan, Jerome. *Understanding Children: Behavior, Motives and Thought*. New York: Harcourt Brace Jovanovich, Ind., 1971.

Kohlberg, Lawrence. *Stages in the Development of Moral Thought and Action*. New York: Holt, Rinehart and Winston, 1969.

Lasker, Judith N. and Borg, Susan. *In Search of Parenthood: Coping with Infertility and High-Tech Conception*. Boston: Beacon Press, 1987.

Laurendeau, M. and Pinard, A. *Causal Thinking in the Child*. New York: International Universities Press, 1962.

Lemke, Sonne. "Identity and Conservation: the Child's Developing Conceptions of Social and Physical Transformation." Unpublished doctoral dissertation, University of California, Berkeley, 1973.

Newman, Judith L, Roberts, Laura R. and Syre, Christine R. (1993) "Concepts of Family Among Children and Adolescents: Effect of Cognitive Level, Gender, and Family Structure." *Developmental Psychology* 29(6), pp. 951-962.

Pederson, David R. and Gilby, Rhonda L. "Children's Concepts of the Family," Chapter Seven in Ashmore, R.D. and Brodzinsky, D. M., *op. cit.*, 1986.

Piaget, Jean. *The Child's Conception of the World*. Totowa, NJ: Littlefield, Adams and Company, 1975.

Piaget, Jean. *The Child's Conception of Physical Causality*. Totowa, NJ: Littlefield, Adams and Company, 1975.

Piaget, Jean. *Judgement and Reasoning in the Child*. Totowa, NJ: Littlefield, Adams and Company, 1968.

Piaget, Jean and Inhelder, Barbel. *The Psychology of the Child.* New York: Basic Books, 1960.

Pomeroy, Wardell B. *Your Child and Sex: a Guide for Parents.* New York: Dell Publishing Company, 1974.

Turiel, Elliot. "Heterogeneity, Inconsistency, and Asynchrony in the Development of Cognitive Structures," in I. Levin (Ed.) *Stage and Structure: Reopening the Debate.* Norwood, NJ: Ablex, 1986.

Turiel, Elliot. "Developmental Processes in the Child's Moral Thinking," in Mussen, P., Langer, J. and Covinton, M. (eds.) *New Directions in Developmental Psychology.* New York: Holt, Rinehart and Winston, 1969.

Watkins, Mary and Fisher, Susan. *Talking with Young Children about Adoption.* New Haven: Yale University Press, 1993.

Wallerstein, Judith and Kelly, Joan Berlin. *Surviving the Breakup: How Children and Parents Cope with Divorce.* New York: Basic Books, 1980.

Resources for Children: Preschool

Gordon, Sol. *Did the Sun Shine Before You Were Born?* Fayetteville, NY: Ed-U Press, 1982.

Koch, Janice. *Our Baby: A Birth and Adoption Story.* Indianapolis: Perspectives Press, 1985.

Schoen, Mark. *Bellybuttons are Navels.* NY: Prometheus Books, 1990.

Stein, Sara Bonnett. *That New Baby.* New York: Walker and Company, 1974.

Vigna, Judith. *Daddy's New Baby.* Niles, IL: Albert Whitman and Company, 1982.

Elementary School-Aged Children

Berman, Claire. *What Am I Doing in a Stepfamily?* Seacaucus, NJ: Lyle Stuart, 1982.

Blank, Joani. *A Kid's First Book about Sex.* Burlingame, CA: Yes Press, 1983.

Boyd, Lizi. *Sam is My Half Brother.* New York: Viking, 1990.

Brown, Laurene Krasny and Brown, Marc. *Dinosaurs Divorce: A Guide for Changing Families.* Boston: Little Brown, 1986.

Cole, Joanna. *How You Were Born.* New York, William Morrow, 1984.

Hauscherr, Rosemarie. *Children and the AIDS Virus: A Book for Children, Parents, and Teachers.* New York: Clarion, 1989.

Lewis, Helen Coale. *All About Families-The Second Time Around.* Atlanta: Peachtree Publishers, 1980.

Newman, Leslea. *Heather Has Two Mommies*. Boston, MA: Alyson Publications, Inc. 1989.

Quackenbush, Marcia and Villareal, Sylvia. *Does AIDS Hurt?* Santa Cruz, CA: Network Publications, 1988.

Schaffer, Patricia. *How Babies and Families are Made (There Is. More Than One Way)*. Berkeley, CA: Tabor Sarah Books, 1988.

Schilling, Sharon and Swan, Jonathon *"My Name is Jonathon (and I Have AIDS),"* Denver: Prickly Pear, 1989.

Stein, Sara Bonnett. *That New Baby.* New York: Walker and Company, 1974.

Stein, Stephanie. *Lucy's Feet.* Indianapolis: Perspectives Press, 1992.

Stenson, Janet S. *Now I Have a Stepparent, And It's Kind of Confusing.* Avon, 1979.

Tax, Meredith. *Families.* New York: Little, Brown, 1981.

Willhoite, Michael. *Daddy's Roommate.* Boston, MA: Alyson Publications, Inc. 1992.

Preadolescents

Calderone, Mary S. and Johnson, Eric W. *The Family Book about Sexuality.* Scranton, PA: Harper Collins, 1990.

Gardner-Loulan, JoAnn, Lopex, Bonnie, and Quackenbush, Marcia. *Period.* Volcano, CA: Volcano Press, 1990.

Gitchel, Sam and Foster, Lorri. *Let's Talk about S-E-X.* Fresno, CA: Planned Parenthood Central California, 1983.

Hynes, Alicia. *Puberty: An Illustrated Manual.* New York: St. Martin's Press: 1989.

Johnson, Eric W. *Love and Sex in Plain Language.* Scranton, PA: Harper Collins, 1985.

Johnson, Eric. W. *People, Love, Sex and Families.* New York: Walker and Company, 1985.

Krementz, Jill. *How It Feels to be Adopted.* New York: Alfred A. Knopf, 1988.

Madaras, Linda. *What's Happening to my Body: For Girls.* New York: New Market Press, 1988.

Madaras, Linda. *What's Happening to my Body: For Boys.* New York: New Market Press, 1988.

Mayle, Peter. *What's Happening to Me?* Secaucus, NJ: Carol Publishing Group, 1975.

For Adolescents:

Bell, Ruth. *Changing Bodies, Changing Lives.* Westminster, MD: Random House, 1987.

Fiedler, Jean and Fiedler, Hal. *Be Smart about Sex.* Hillside, NJ: Enslow Publishers, Inc. 1990.

Getzoff, Ann & McClenahan, Carolyn. *Stepkids: A Survival Guide for Teenagers in Stepfamilies.* New York: Walter and Co., 1984.

Heron, Ann. *One Teenager in 10: Writings by Gay and Lesbian Youth.* Boston, MA: Alyson Publications, Inc. 1983.

McCoy, Kathy and Wibbelsman, Charles. *The New Teenage Body Book.* Los Angeles: Price Stern Sloan, Inc., 1987.

For Adults:

Bell, Ruth and Wildflower, Leni Zeiger. *Talking With Your Teenager: A Book for Parents.* New York: Random House, 1982.

Bernstein, Anne C. *Yours, Mine, and Ours: How Families Change When Remarried Parents Have a Child Together.* New York: W. W. Norton, 1990.

Brodzinsky, David M., Schechter, Marshall D., and Henig, Robin Marantz. *Being Adopted: The Lifelong Search for Self.* New York: Doubleday, 1992.

Calderone, Mary S. and Johnson, Eric W. *The Family Book about Sexuality.* Scranton, PA: Harper Collins, 1990.

Cassell, Carol. *Straight from the Heart: How to Talk to Your Teenagers about Love and Sex.* New York: Fireside, 1987.

Cooper, Susan L. and Glazer. Ellen S. Beyond Infertility: *The New Paths to Parenthood*. New York: Lexington, 1994.

Glazer, Ellen Sarasohn. *The Long Awaited Stork: A Guide to Parenting after Infertility*. Lexington, MA: Lexington Books, 1990.

Goldman, Ronald and Goldman, Juliette. *Show Me Yours: Understanding Children's Sexuality*. New York, Penguin, 1988.

Hynes, Angela. *Puberty: An Illustrated Manual for Parents and Daughters*. New York: Tor, 1990.

Johnston, Patricia Irwin. *Adopting After Infertility*. Indianapolis: Perspectives Press, 1992.

Keshet, Jamie Kelem. *Love and Power in the Stepfamily: A Practical Guide*. New York: McGraw-Hill, 1987.

Leight, Lynn. *Raising Sexually Healthy Children: A Loving Guide for Parents, Teachers, and Caregivers*. New York: Rawson Associates,1989.

Martin, April. *Lesbian and Gay Parenting*. New York: Harper Collins, 1993.

Stark, Patty. *Sex is More than a Plumbing Lesson: A Parent's Guide to Sexuality Education for Infants through the Teen Years*. Dallas: Preston Hollow Enterprises, 1990.

Strasburger, Victor. *Getting Your Kids to Say "No" in the 90's When You Said "Yes" in the 60's*. New York: Fireside, 1993.

Sullivan, Susan K. and Kawiak, Matthew A. *Parents Talk Love: The Catholic Family Handbook about Sexuality*. Mahwah, NJ: Paulist Press,1985.

Visher, Emily B. and Visher, John S. *How to Win as a Stepfamily*. Second Edition. New York: Brunner/Mazel, 1991.

Watkins, Mary and Fisher, Susan. *Talking with Young Children about Adoption*. New Haven: Yale University Press, 1993.

*I*ndex

*A*bout the Author

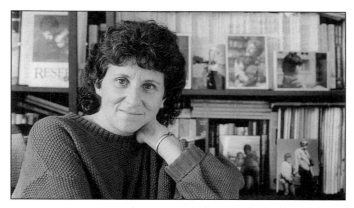

Anne C. Bernstein, Ph.D. is a Professor of Psychology at the Wright Institute in Berkeley, CA, where she is a practicing family psychologist. She is the author of *Yours, Mine, and Ours: How Families Change When Remarried Parents Have a Child Together* (Charles Scribner's Sons, 1989; W. W. Norton, 1990) and is a frequent contributor to professional books and journals and to *Parents Magazine*. Dr. Bernstein has served on the Board of Directors of the American Family Therapy Academy and the Stepfamily Association of America, for which she chairs the Clinical Committee. She lives with her husband and son in Berkeley, California.

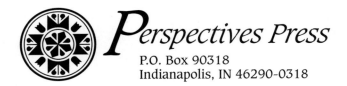

Perspectives Press
P.O. Box 90318
Indianapolis, IN 46290-0318

Since 1982 Perspectives Press has focused exclusively on infertility, adoption, and related reproductive and child welfare issues. Our purpose is to promote understanding of these issues and to educate and sensitize those personally experiencing these life situations, professionals who work in these fields and the public at large. Our titles are never duplicative or competitive with material already available through other publishers. We seek to find and fill only niches which are empty. In addition to this book, our current titles include:

For Adults

Perspectives on a Grafted Tree

Understanding: A Guide to Impaired Fertility for Family and Friends

Sweet Grapes: How to Stop Being Infertile and Start Living Again

Residential Treatment: A Tapestry of Many Therapies

A Child's Journey Through Placement

Adopting after Infertility

Taking Charge of Infertility

For Children

Our Baby: A Birth and Adoption Story

The Mulberry Bird: Story of an Adoption

Real for Sure Sister

Filling in the Blanks: A Guided Look at Growing Up Adopted

Where the Sun Kisses the Sea

William Is My Brother

Lucy's Feet